Contents

Introduction 5
Chapter 1 All About Allergies 9
Chapter 2 Reduce Your Child's Risk 19
Chapter 3 Allergy Symptoms and Diseases 27
Chapter 4 Getting a Diagnosis 39
Chapter 5 Avoiding Common Allergens 49
Chapter 6 Coping with Food Allergies 57
Chapter 7 Allergy Treatments 67
Chapter 8 Dealing with Medical Emergencies 77
Chapter 9 Using Complementary Therapies 87
Chapter 10 Raising a Confident Child 95
Chapter 11 Allergies at School 103
Chapter 12 Living with Allergies 111
Help List 119

Introduction

Britain is in the grip of an allergy epidemic. The incidence of allergy is amongst the highest in the world, with one in four people suffering from an allergy at some point in their lifetime. According to the House of Lords Science and Technology Committee's Sixth Report on Allergy in July 2007, cases of asthma, eczema and hayfever have tripled in the last 20 years, with nearly 40% of children now affected. Some children are suffering from more than one allergic condition at a time. Most worryingly, there has been a dramatic rise in the number of children with serious food allergies. Peanut allergy has shown the largest rise, by 117% in just four years (between 2001 and 2005).

If your child has been diagnosed with an allergy, it's natural to be overwhelmed with questions. Will you be able to identify, and avoid, all of the triggers? What's the best way to treat your child's symptoms? Could your child have a severe reaction? Will your child grow out of it? What do you tell your child's school?

As the mother of a child with peanut allergy, and another with hayfever, I know how daunting it can be when you're given the initial diagnosis. Some families find it very difficult to obtain specialist help because there are very few paediatric allergy specialists in the UK, which adds to the worry and despair.

This book is for all parents who suspect their child has an allergy or want to prevent allergies. The information is based on current clinical guidance and the latest medical research, with practical tips and coping strategies to guide you through the allergy maze. It can't, and shouldn't, replace the advice from your child's healthcare professionals, but it will hopefully give you essential background information and reassurance.

If you want to learn more about allergies in children, it helps to have a basic understanding of what an allergy is. Chapter 1 looks at the background to allergies – what happens when you have an allergy and common triggers. Chapter 2 looks at the current research into allergy prevention, with guidance for pregnant women and parents of young children. Chapters 3 and 4 cover identifying allergy symptoms and the importance of seeking a diagnosis, as

> 'Most worryingly, there has been a dramatic rise in the number of children with serious food allergies. Peanut allergy has shown the largest rise, by 117% in just four years.'

well as a brief guide to common allergy tests. Once you have established what your child is allergic to, you can learn how to avoid common allergy triggers in chapter 5 with some simple practical measures.

If your child has food allergies, chapter 6 will give you advice on avoiding culprit foods, consulting a dietitian and shopping for food so that you can keep your child safe at all times, even when you are away from home. Chapters 7, 8 and 9 cover the use of allergy medicines, dealing with medical emergencies and choosing complementary therapies so that you can learn more about keeping your child's allergies under control.

It can be a shock when your child is first diagnosed with an allergy, especially if it's potentially life-threatening. Chapter 10 can help you deal with your emotions and give you guidance on explaining allergies to your child or teenager so that they can begin to take some control over their symptoms. Chapter 11 is aimed at parents of children at pre-school, nursery or school, with advice on avoiding their allergy triggers, what to tell their teachers and putting together a management plan.

Some children do eventually grow out of their allergies. If your child's allergy continues into late childhood and the teenage years, it's important that they don't grow up feeling any different to their peers. There's no denying that having an allergy can affect all aspects of your child's welfare, from their growth and development through to their education and social wellbeing, but this only happens if you let it.

Chapter 12 covers activities and celebrations such as holidays, days out, Christmas and birthday parties. These needn't be a chore with careful planning. And the good news is that if you can learn how to manage your child's symptoms successfully and reduce the risk of flare-ups, you can stop the allergy from taking over not only your child's life but that of the whole family.

The help list at the end of the book provides you with the contact details of the organisations, charities and product suppliers mentioned in the book.

Disclaimer

This book is for general information on childhood allergies and isn't intended to replace professional medical advice. If you suspect that your child has an allergy, it is important to consult a healthcare professional and obtain a proper diagnosis. If your child has been diagnosed with an allergy, you should follow the allergy avoidance and management advice given to you by your child's GP and allergy consultant.

All the information in this book was correct at the time of going to press. National guidelines and recommendations can change, so it is important to check with your child's GP and allergy consultant before acting on any of the information in this book.

Chapter One

All About Allergies

According to the national charity Allergy UK, allergies affect one in four of the UK population. Each year numbers increase by 5%, with as many as half of those affected being children.

To understand why your child has an allergy or is at risk of an allergy and the best way to treat it, it helps if you understand how an allergy occurs and what makes the symptoms appear. If allergies run in your family, learning about the risk factors may help to reduce the chance that your child, or any children you have in the future, will develop an allergy themselves.

What is an allergy?

There's a lot of dispute over the meaning of the word 'allergy', and people use it in various ways. These days, most allergy specialists use the word 'allergy' to describe an over-reaction by the immune system to a substance that is harmless to non-allergic people.

The immune system protects the body from invasion by bacteria, viruses and anything else that threatens its wellbeing, e.g. cancer cells. Normally, it can tell the difference between self and non-self (i.e. the body's cells versus a virus) and harmless and harmful, e.g. dust versus bacteria. However, in allergic people the immune system can't recognise that some substances (allergens such as pollen or dust) are harmless, so it seeks to destroy them instead. This can cause a wide range of symptoms from sneezing or itchy skin to anaphylactic shock.

> 'There is considerable confusion amongst the general public over what an allergy actually is and what sort of symptoms can be caused by an allergy.'
>
> Professor Gideon Lack, Head of Children's Allergy Service, Guy's and St Thomas' NHS Foundation Trust and Professor of Paediatric Allergy, King's College London.

Types of allergic reactions

There are two main types of allergic reaction: IgE-mediated reactions and non-IgE mediated reactions. IgE (allergy antibodies) are produced during most allergic reactions when the body comes into contact with a specific allergen.

IgE-mediated reactions (true allergies)

- These account for around 90% of true food allergies.
- The reactions involve the over-production of IgE antibodies.
- They tend to be immediate, so the symptoms appear straightaway and the allergen is usually obvious.
- Only very tiny amounts of an allergen are needed to trigger a reaction.
- Examples include immediate urticaria (also called hives, nettle rash or welts) or anaphylactic shock, often in response to food allergens.

Non-IgE mediated reactions

- Doctors still don't fully understand non-IgE mediated reactions but think that these reactions involve other immune system cells such as T helper 1 (Th1) cells.
- The reactions are usually triggered by larger amounts of a food or substance.
- It can take 24 to 48 hours for the symptoms to appear.
- These reactions are usually more difficult to diagnose than IgE-mediated allergies because the trigger isn't obvious.
- Examples include atopic eczema, contact dermatitis and coeliac disease (gluten intolerance).

Food intolerance

- Many hypersensitivity reactions to foods are not due to an allergy at all and don't even involve the immune system. These are called food intolerances, and often occur because that person doesn't have a particular enzyme which is needed to break down a particular food substance, e.g. lactose in milk.
- The symptoms may be similar to those of a true allergic reaction, although they rarely progress to anaphylaxis.
- For more information see chapter 6.

IgE sensitisation

A true allergic reaction always involves the production of IgE antibodies (immunoglobulins). Antibodies are produced by specialist white blood cells called B-cells. They bind to bacteria, viruses, etc and there are several different types, each with a slightly different job in the immune system. The main role of IgE antibodies is to defend the body against parasites, such as ringworm, which are larger than bacteria and viruses. However, IgE antibodies also attach to allergens.

The first time the immune system is exposed to an allergen, this doesn't cause any symptoms in the allergic person. Instead, B-cells produce small amounts of IgE which then stay in the bloodstream. This initial exposure is called 'sensitisation' and basically gets the body ready for another attack, should one occur. Research shows that most people are sensitised to allergens in the first two years of their life.

The next time this person comes into contact with the same allergen, their immune system will now mount an attack, perceiving the substance to be harmful. Again, IgE antibodies are produced, but this time they are produced much faster and in much larger quantities. They attach first to the allergen and then to a type of white blood cell called a mast cell. The mast cell releases histamine and other chemicals that trigger inflammation and allergy symptoms.

Common allergens

Allergens can enter your child's body through their nose, mouth, skin, eyes and airways, and they vary from person to person. Hayfever can be triggered by different allergens (e.g. grass and tree pollens) in different people, or by several allergens in one person.

Most allergic disorders can be triggered by more than one allergen. For example, eczema can be triggered by food, house dust mites or chemicals on the skin.

Allergens always contain protein which forms an essential part of most living organisms, as well as a lot of the food we eat. Some substances that don't contain protein, e.g. medicines like penicillin, can also provoke an allergic reaction as they bind to proteins when they enter the body.

According to the charity Allergy UK, the most common allergens in the UK are:

- House dust mites.
- Grass and tree pollens.
- Cats.
- Dogs.
- Insects, e.g. wasps and bees.
- Milk.
- Eggs.
- Peanuts.

Less common allergens are:

- Tree nuts.
- Fruit.
- Latex.

See chapter 5 for advice on avoiding common allergens.

'Allergens vary from person to person. Hayfever can be triggered by different allergens in different people, or by several allergens in one person.'

Cross-reactivity

Each IgE antibody works like a key so that it attaches (binds) – and therefore reacts – to a specific allergen only. This is why the antibodies are known as specific-IgE.

Very occasionally, IgE antibodies bind to more than one allergen because the proteins in these allergens are very similar. This is called a cross-reaction. Here are some examples:

- Many people who are allergic to house dust mites also react to cockroaches, which can trigger asthma.
- A person who is allergic to latex may react to particular foods e.g. bananas, avocados and kiwi fruit.
- People with hayfever may react to apples.

Allergy symptoms

Allergy symptoms may appear straightaway after the exposure to an allergen or may be delayed for several hours. They can last for only a few minutes or may last for days.

The symptoms aren't caused by the allergens themselves. They are triggered by the chemicals released by the immune system during the allergic reaction. Different chemicals may be produced which is why allergy symptoms are so varied. The two main chemicals are:

- Histamine: this triggers the classic immediate symptoms of allergy, such as sneezing, itching and a rash. In large amounts it also triggers a drop in blood pressure, which causes anaphylaxis.
- Leukotrienes: these cause prolonged symptoms like airway narrowing and swelling, leading to shortness of breath and wheezing. They are often associated with asthma.

Long term (chronic) allergy symptoms, like a persistent blocked or runny nose, may be caused by white blood cells called T helper 2 (Th2) cells which release other chemicals called cytokines and chemokines.

Allergy treatments

Anti-allergy medicines work in different ways to stop the immune reaction.

- Steroid drugs dampen down the whole immune system.
- Antihistamines block histamine production.
- Anti-leukotrienes block leukotrienes and are used in asthma.
- Sodium cromoglicate stops mast cells releasing allergy chemicals.

For more information on allergy medicines see chapter 7.

Family history and allergies

> 'Children get half of their genes from their mother and half from their father. A child's risk of allergy is increased if one or both of their parents are affected.'

Allergies tend to run in families.

- Children get half of their genes from their mother and half from their father.
- A child's risk of an allergy is increased if one or both of their parents are affected.
- According to the British Society for Allergy and Clinical Immunology (BSACI), a child who has a mother with an allergy has a 60% chance of developing an allergy themselves – this rises to an 80% chance if both their parents have allergies.
- Children may not suffer from the same allergy symptoms as their parents. You or your partner may have rhinitis, for example, while your child has asthma or eczema.

What is atopy?

If your child is prone to IgE-mediated allergic reactions, they are considered to be atopic. They will have inherited the tendency to produce large amounts of IgE antibodies in response to low doses of allergens. A child who is not prone to allergies will have only small amounts of IgE in their body.

People who are atopic are more likely to develop allergic conditions like eczema, allergic asthma and hayfever. However, not everyone who is atopic will develop an allergic disorder, and some people may not develop an allergy until later in life. There are also some people who have positive IgE blood test results but never experience any allergy symptoms.

Your environment and allergies

Allergy experts don't yet understand why allergies have become so common. It's clear that a person's family history is important. However, according to the House of Lords Science and Technology Committee's Sixth Report on Allergy, the rise in allergies can't be explained simply by genetics as the genetic background of the whole population hasn't changed that significantly over the last 50 years. It now seems that environmental factors, e.g. how people live, also have an important part to play.

There are various theories on how a child's environment affects their risk of allergies, but none of the evidence is conclusive. The following theories are taken from the House of Lords' report.

The hygiene hypothesis

In the 1980s, British epidemiologist David Strachan proposed that children who are exposed to poor hygiene and increased infections in early life have less risk of allergies. There has been a lot of support for this hypothesis. For example, pregnant women and children who grow up on farms have less risk of allergies and asthma than those living in other rural areas. However, there are also studies suggesting that early infections can actually trigger allergies, so there's still a lot of research to do.

'The rise in allergies can't be explained simply by genetics as the genetic background of the whole population hasn't changed that significantly over the last 50 years.'

Diet in pregnancy and early childhood

The mother's diet during pregnancy and a child's diet in their early years also seem to be important in determining a child's risk of allergies. Exclusive breastfeeding in the first three months of life seems to offer the most protection. The theory that early exposure to allergens such as peanuts may offer some protection is now being questioned (see chapter 2).

Allergen exposure

Another theory is that children these days are exposed to more allergens, increasing their chance of becoming sensitised. However, allergy avoidance doesn't necessarily prevent allergies. For example, reducing house dust mite levels in the home doesn't always reduce symptoms in children with dust allergy. There's also evidence that children who live with cats and dogs from an early age are less likely to develop allergies.

Tobacco smoke

Children living with parents who smoke are more prone to wheezing, asthma and respiratory symptoms. However, the report from the House of Lords states that research hasn't yet found any specific link between smoking and allergy development.

Indoor environment

Damp housing conditions can cause house dust mites and mould to thrive, all of which can make asthma worse. Various chemicals in the air, such as nitrogen oxides from gas cookers, can also trigger asthma symptoms. However, there's no evidence that a child's indoor environment triggers their allergy to develop in the first place.

> 'The mother's diet during pregnancy and the diet in early childhood seem to be important in determining a child's risk of allergies.'

Pollution levels

Exposure to high levels of pollution in cities from cars and other vehicles may worsen respiratory allergy symptoms. Some air pollutants make pollen more likely to trigger reactions in susceptible people.

Summing Up

- An allergy occurs when the immune system over-reacts to a substance that is harmless to people without that particular allergy.
- True allergic reactions involve IgE antibodies.
- All allergens contain protein or bind to protein when they enter the body.
- Allergy symptoms are triggered by chemicals produced during an allergic reaction.
- Allergies usually run in families. Children who are prone to IgE-mediated reactions are called 'atopic'.
- There are various theories about why allergies are becoming increasingly common, but there's still a lot of ongoing research.

Chapter Two

Reduce Your Child's Risk

It's natural to want the best for your child – especially when it comes to their health. If allergies run in your family, there are some steps you can take to help reduce your child's risk of developing an allergy, either before you have a baby or while your child is still very young.

It's important to remember though that not all children from atopic families will develop allergies – and some babies will develop allergies no matter how many precautions you take. The research into preventing allergies in children is ongoing and there's no conclusive evidence that any of the following steps will definitely work. If your child does develop an allergy, remember that any precautions you have taken may have made the symptoms less severe than they would otherwise have been.

Quitting smoking

Stopping smoking isn't easy, but it's one of the best things you can do, not only for your health but for your child's health too. Babies born to mothers who smoke tend to have smaller airways, making them more susceptible to breathing problems, asthma and allergies, and they are at a higher risk of cot death. Smoking can also increase the risk of complications during labour and the risk of miscarriage, premature delivery or stillbirth.

Breathing in second-hand smoke is also harmful as tobacco smoke contains over 4,000 toxic chemicals. According to the NHS Smokefree website (www.smokefree.nhs.uk), children who grow up in homes where one or both parents smoke are more prone to:

- Coughs, colds and other respiratory infections.

'It's important to remember that not all children from atopic families will develop allergies – and some babies will develop allergies no matter how many precautions you take.'

- Glue ear (a build-up of fluid in the middle ear) which can lead to partial deafness.
- Hospitalisation for a serious respiratory infection.
- Asthma and asthma attacks.
- Meningitis.

Ways to quit

Ideally, you should quit smoking before you conceive, but giving up at any time during or after pregnancy can benefit you and your child. You are four times more likely to quit if you use one of the free NHS support services as well as stop smoking medicines like nicotine patches or gum.

- If you want to quit smoking, speak to a pharmacist about nicotine replacement products. If you are pregnant, it should be safe for you to use these products but check with your GP first.
- You can get stop smoking medicines on prescription, so it doesn't have to cost a fortune.
- Ask your friends, family and work colleagues not to smoke around you – or, even better, persuade them to quit too.
- If you fail at first, keep trying.
- Get some professional support.

For free smoking cessation advice, you can call the NHS Smoking Helpline, the NHS Pregnancy Smoking Helpline or Quitline, run by the stop smoking charity Quit. See the help list at the back of this book for details.

Breastfeeding benefits

The World Health Organisation (WHO) recommends that babies are exclusively breastfed until they reach six months, although any amount of breastfeeding can benefit a baby's health. Breastfeeding gives babies under six months all the nutrients they need and protects them against infections by passing on the mother's protective antibodies. Breastfeeding is good for bonding with your baby too.

Research shows that breastfed babies are less prone than bottle fed babies to:

- Asthma.
- Eczema.
- Ear infections.
- Obesity.
- Infections of the digestive system.

Mothers who breastfeed are at a lower risk of:

- Breast cancer.
- Ovarian cancer.
- Weak bones (osteoporosis) in later life.

See the NHS breastfeeding website (www.breastfeeding.nhs.uk) for more information.

Get some support

Women stop breastfeeding for various reasons, including the baby rejecting the breast or painful breasts or nipples. Others stop for personal reasons, such as juggling other children or going back to work. Getting the right support is therefore crucial.

Your midwife, health visitor or GP will be able to help with breastfeeding problems. You can also contact various organisations for support and information, including the National Childbirth Trust (NCT), the National Breastfeeding Helpline or the Association of Breastfeeding Mothers. See help list for details.

'There is some evidence suggesting that exclusive breastfeeding for the first three months of life reduces the child's risk of developing allergies. However, there's no firm evidence that exclusive breastfeeding beyond the first three months reduces allergies.'

Professor Gideon Lack, Head of Children's Allergy Service, Guy's and St Thomas' NHS Foundation Trust and Professor of Paediatric Allergy, King's College London.

Bottle feeding

If you can't or don't want to breastfeed, you shouldn't feel guilty. Not all women choose to breastfeed from birth, and some women can't breastfeed for the recommended length of time. Infant formula milks are specially formulated so they can be offered as an alternative to breastfeeding.

Low risk babies

- Use cow's milk based infant formula milks until your baby is one year, unless advised otherwise by your health visitor or GP. Cow's milk based follow-on infant formulas are suitable from six months.
- From one year, your child can drink full-fat cow's milk. Don't give your child semi-skimmed cow's milk until two years, or skimmed or 1% milk until five years.
- Goat and sheep milks are not suitable until one year as they don't contain the right balance of nutrients.
- All milks should be pasteurised.

High risk babies

- If your child has a sibling or one or both parents with an allergy, they may be prescribed infant formula milks that carry less risk of allergy than standard cow's milk formulas. Called extensively hydrolysed casein infant formulas, these are specially treated to break down the protein that triggers cow's milk allergy.
- Partially hydrolysed infant formulas still contain some cow's milk protein and aren't suitable for babies who have been diagnosed with milk allergy. However, there's some evidence that using these milks can reduce the risk of some allergic diseases (but not eczema) in high risk babies.
- You should only use soya-based infant formulas on the advice of your GP or health visitor, as babies who are allergic to cow's milk may react to soya as well.

Weaning onto solids

The Department of Health currently recommends that you shouldn't wean your baby onto solid foods until they are six months (26 weeks), whether they are breastfed or bottle fed. By around six months, your baby's natural iron stores run out and they can't get enough supplies from milk. The Food Standards Agency (FSA) suggests that parents introduce solid foods in four stages so that by the time your baby is one year they should be eating a normal, healthy and varied diet.

Some parents want to wean earlier than six months, but current Department of Health guidelines say that 17 weeks is the earliest suitable age. Before this babies aren't physically ready to cope with solid food and their digestive and immune systems may not be mature enough. If your baby was born prematurely, you should discuss the timing of weaning with your GP or health visitor as this will depend on your baby's development.

Suitable foods

Many foods aren't suitable for babies under six months, including eggs both raw and cooked, fish, shellfish, liver, soft or unpasteurised cheeses and gluten containing foods, e.g. wheat, barley or rye. You shouldn't add salt to your baby's food as this can harm their kidneys, while sugar can encourage a sweet tooth and contribute to tooth decay. Honey isn't suitable for babies until 12 months as very occasionally it can carry a type of bacteria called *Clostridium botulinum* that can make young babies very ill.

The FSA can provide good general advice on the weaning stages and feeding babies with allergies. However, if your child is at a high risk of allergies, speak to your GP, health visitor or allergy consultant. You may be given specific advice on introducing certain foods, e.g. egg, milk, soya and gluten-containing foods, into your child's diet. If your child already has allergies, you will probably have to take extra precautions.

'The FSA can provide good general advice on the weaning stages and feeding babies with allergies. However, if your child is at a high risk of allergies, speak to your GP, health visitor or allergy consultant.'

Peanut avoidance...

Peanuts are one of the most common food allergens in the UK and can cause severe reactions, including anaphylaxis. At the time of writing this book, the Department of Health advises that peanuts should be avoided during pregnancy, while breastfeeding and until your child is three years if there's a close family history of any atopic disease, e.g. asthma, eczema or hayfever.

This advice is based on research showing that avoiding peanuts may stop a baby's immune system from becoming sensitised to peanut protein, and therefore may prevent allergic reactions as the child gets older.

If you follow this advice, your child will need to avoid contact with all peanut-containing foods as well as some cosmetics and toiletries (e.g. nipple creams) that contain arachis oil (oil extracted from peanuts). Some parents choose not to give their children any nuts, not just peanuts, until they reach three years. If you don't have a family history of allergies, you don't need to follow this advice. However, children shouldn't have any whole nuts until they reach five years, due to the risk of choking.

... or peanut consumption

In some countries in Africa and Asia, there's no such thing as peanut allergy, even though children consume large amounts of peanuts from an early age. In December 2008, the Food Standards Agency's Committee on Toxicity reviewed the research available and found no clear indication that exposure to, or avoidance of, peanuts in pregnancy and early life provides protection. The FSA no longer recommends peanut avoidance, although there's no evidence that it does children any harm. The Department of Health is now looking into the issue, but until there's new official guidance it's important that you continue with peanut avoidance if allergies run in your family.

The LEAP (Learning Early About Peanut Allergy) study, which is based at the Evelina Children's Hospital, Guy's and St Thomas' NHS Foundation Trust in London, is one of the research studies looking at whether peanut avoidance or peanut exposure puts children at risk of peanut allergy. The research is still in its early stages.

> 'To eat, or not to eat? That's the ultimate question in the prevention of food allergy. Currently the evidence is inconclusive. In order to understand the best way to prevent peanut allergy, it's necessary to do a proper study comparing both dietary strategies.'
>
> Professor Gideon Lack, Head of Children's Allergy Service, Guy's and St Thomas' NHS Foundation Trust and Professor of Paediatric Allergy, King's College London.

Your baby's skincare routine

According to the National Eczema Society, atopic eczema begins in the first year of life in around 60% of children with eczema. Research shows that susceptible people carry a specific faulty gene which means that they have a damaged skin barrier. This makes their skin dry out easily, especially if they use soap or detergents, increasing their risk of eczema and other dry skin conditions.

While there currently isn't any evidence to show that how you look after your baby's skin will affect their risk of eczema, it's still important to prevent dry patches and irritation.

Essential tips

- Don't use soap or baby wipes on babies under one month – plain water and cotton wool is sufficient.
- Once your baby is a few weeks old, use specially formulated baby products that are suitable for sensitive skin – but use them sparingly.
- Avoid products that bubble or lather, as these may be more likely to trigger a reaction by stripping your baby's skin of its natural oils.
- Choose sensitive baby wipes that are alcohol-free and fragrance-free, but stop using them if they irritate your baby's skin.
- If your baby reacts to a product, don't use it again and seek advice from your GP or health visitor as soon as possible.
- Babies don't usually need a bath more than once or twice a week, as they don't tend to get dirty until they are crawling. Topping and tailing with cotton wool is adequate on the other days.

Skincare advice is available from the British Skin Foundation and the National Eczema Society. See help list for details.

'If eczema is in your family, it's sensible to avoid using soap products and to wash and moisturise with emollients from an early age.'

Margaret Cox, chief executive of the National Eczema Society.

Summing Up

- If allergies run in your family, there are steps you can take to reduce your child's risk of developing one.
- Smoking during pregnancy can increase the risk of a baby developing asthma or breathing problems.
- If allergies run in your family, you may wish to avoid peanuts during pregnancy and while breastfeeding, and for children up to the age of three years.
- Breastfeeding protects children from allergies, obesity and infections.
- Bottle fed babies at a high risk of allergies can be given extensively hydrolysed infant formulas.
- When you wean your baby onto solid food (from six months), introduce only small amounts of common food allergens, e.g. eggs and cow's milk, and give them one at a time. See your GP or health visitor for more information.
- Look after your baby's skin carefully to prevent it from drying out.

'If allergies run in your family, there are steps you can take to reduce your child's risk of developing one.'

Chapter Three

Allergy Symptoms and Diseases

Allergies cause a wide range of symptoms and affect children in different ways. When your child experiences the symptoms for the first time, you may not actually realise that they have had an allergic reaction. This is because many allergy symptoms are similar to those of other common childhood infections or conditions.

Typical symptoms

Your child may have just one allergy symptom or several. The symptoms are often similar for different allergic diseases and can change over time. General allergy symptoms include:

- A runny nose.
- Sneezing.
- A blocked or stuffy nose.
- Itchy eyes, ears, lips, throat or roof of the mouth.
- Coughing, especially at night.
- Wheezing and shortness of breath.
- Rashes.
- Tiredness.
- Redness in the face.

Some of these symptoms can be caused by other illnesses too, so it's important to see your GP if you are worried about them.

Hidden symptoms

Sometimes an allergy can cause symptoms that aren't typical, especially in children, making them less easy to spot. These include:

- Headaches.
- Unexplained irritability.
- Nausea.
- Itching with no signs of a rash.
- Digestive upsets.
- Hyperactivity.

If your child has any unusual, severe or persistent symptoms, it's important to get them checked out by your GP. They may be signs of an allergy but could also be something completely different. For example, persistent or recurrent diarrhoea may be due to a problem with their digestive system.

Recognising allergic children

There are some physical signs that can alert an allergy doctor to a child with allergies before they do any allergy tests. These include:

- Unhealthy, pale complexion. Many children with multiple allergies are also small for their age.
- Allergic shiners. These dark circles under the eyes look like the beginnings of a black eye or smudged mascara, or you may just assume your child isn't getting enough sleep. But they are more likely to be due to an increased blood flow near your child's sinuses.
- Creases under the eyelids. Called Dennie-Morgan lines, these are associated with nose-related and chest-related allergies in young children.

'Jessie's symptoms can be mild (like a red itchy rash on her face or at her eczema points) or much more severe. Even the bad reactions vary each time – her face may puff up or she may be persistently sick.'

Gail Flaum, whose six-year-old daughter has eczema and multiple allergies (including egg, nut, chocolate and dust).

- Allergic or 'nasal' salute. Children with a constant runny nose tend to rub their noses upwards with the palm of their hand. This can also lead to a crease across the bridge of the nose.
- Pulling funny faces. If a child's nose, ears or eyes are itchy, they may twitch or wiggle their face. Some children also sniff constantly.
- Dry, rough skin. This is particularly common on the cheeks, upper arms and chest, as well as in the creases of the elbows and behind the knees.
- Poor attention span. Children with glue ear may have difficulty hearing, which can lead to poor concentration.

Classical allergic diseases

These are the main allergic (atopic) diseases that affect children.

Allergic rhinitis

Allergic rhinitis affects over 20% of the UK population, according to the 'British Society for Allergy and Clinical Immunology (BASCI) guidelines for the management of allergic and non-allergic rhinitis' (published in the medical journal *Clinical and Experimental Allergy* in 2008).

Symptoms:

- A blocked and/or runny nose.
- Sneezing.
- Itching.
- Streaming eyes.
- Sometimes asthma.

If the symptoms occur throughout the year (called perennial allergic rhinitis), they may be mistaken for a persistent cold. Symptoms that occur in specific seasons are called seasonal allergic rhinitis or, more commonly, hayfever. Eye symptoms are called allergic conjunctivitis.

'If your child has any unusual, severe or persistent symptoms, it's important to get them checked out by your GP.'

Common triggers:

Perennial allergic rhinitis is usually triggered by house dust mites or animals. Hayfever is usually triggered by pollen (mainly from grass, trees or weeds) or fungal spores. Allergic conjunctivitis is caused by allergens like pollen or dust irritating the membranes of the eye. It's uncomfortable and irritating and both eyes are usually affected.

Allergic asthma

According to Asthma UK, one in 11 children in the UK now has asthma. Asthma affects the airways, the small tubes that carry air in and out of the lungs. If the airways become irritated, e.g. by an allergen, they can become narrower and inflamed. This triggers asthma symptoms.

Symptoms:

According to the 'British Guideline on the Management of Asthma', produced by the British Thoracic Society and the Scottish Intercollegiate Guidelines Network in May 2008, asthma in children causes:

- Recurrent wheezing.
- Coughing.
- Difficulty breathing.
- Chest tightness.

These symptoms are often worse at night and in the early morning. In severe cases, an asthma attack, the child can't breathe enough oxygen into their lungs.

Common triggers:

Allergic triggers include house dust mites, pollen, moulds, pets and, very occasionally, food allergies. Some children have non-allergic triggers too, such as viral infections, exercise, certain drugs and exposure to fumes or tobacco smoke.

Atopic eczema

According to the National Eczema Society (NES), atopic eczema affects one in five children in the UK. It generally develops in the first six to 12 months of life.

Symptoms:

Eczema looks different in each child, but mild cases usually cause dry, scaly, red and itchy patches of skin. The intense itching is particularly distressing for children, and young babies may rub their faces on their cot sheets or clothes. In severe cases the skin may weep, crust and bleed, leaving it prone to infections. According to the NES, atopic eczema usually starts on the face and scalp but often spreads to other areas, especially inside the elbows and behind the knees. In severe cases it can cover most of the body.

Common triggers:

The main allergic triggers include house dust mites, pets or some foods, especially egg. Eczema can also be triggered by other factors, such as stress, soaps, detergents and infections.

Urticaria

According to the British Association of Dermatologists, around one in five people in the UK will experience urticaria, also called hives, nettle rash or welts, at some point in their lifetime.

Symptoms:

Urticaria causes itchy red swellings (weals) on the surface of the skin. Acute symptoms can last for up to six weeks, while chronic urticaria can last for several months. Angioedema is a much more severe form, causing large raised bumps under the surface of the skin as well as puffiness around the eyes and lips.

'In a third to a half of children, the eczema is associated with an underlying food allergy. Young children with significant eczema should therefore undergo allergy testing at the time of expansive dietary weaning.'

Dr George Du Toit, consultant in paediatric allergy at St Thomas' Hospital.

Common triggers:

The cause is often never found, although food allergies, medicines, e.g. penicillin, and viral infections are possible triggers.

Oral allergy syndrome

According to Allergy UK, oral allergy syndrome is becoming increasingly common, with as many as one in 20 children affected. It's a form of cross-reaction where people who are allergic to birch or hazel pollens or latex also react to some foods (e.g. fruits or nuts).

Symptoms:

Swelling, tingling or itching on the lips, mouth, tongue or throat. The symptoms usually start immediately upon eating the culprit food. General symptoms like urticaria, rhinitis or asthma may also develop.

Common triggers:

Various fruits, including apples, cherries, peaches and plums, and nuts like hazelnuts or walnuts.

Food allergies

According to the Anaphylaxis Campaign, food allergies affect around one in 17 children, with one in 70 suffering from peanut allergy.

Symptoms:

These range from localised rashes to life-threatening anaphylaxis and can affect different parts of the body, e.g. skin rashes, tickly mouth, tongue or throat, abdominal pain, diarrhoea or wheezing.

Common triggers:

The most common food allergens in the UK are:

- Peanuts.
- Tree nuts, e.g. almonds, hazelnuts or cashews.
- Sesame seeds.
- Eggs.
- Cow's milk.
- Shellfish, e.g. prawns.
- Fish.

New allergens (e.g. mustard or kiwi fruit) have also been reported.

See chapter 6 for more in-depth information on food allergies.

Anaphylaxis

Anaphylaxis is a severe allergic reaction that affects the whole body. It's caused by the sudden release of large amounts of allergy chemicals, especially histamine, in response to a specific trigger. Even tiny amounts of allergens can trigger a reaction in susceptible people.

Your child is at high risk if:

- They have experienced a bad allergic reaction in the past.
- They have previously reacted to a very tiny amount of allergen, as a larger amount could trigger more severe symptoms.

Symptoms:

These include:

- Changes in your child's heart rate.
- Swelling of the throat or mouth.
- Severe asthma.
- Difficulty breathing, swallowing or speaking.
- Sudden weakness (drop in blood pressure).

> 'Anaphylaxis, or anaphylactic shock, involves several systems of the body and can be fatal if it's not treated immediately.'
>
> Dr George Du Toit, consultant in paediatric allergy at St Thomas' Hospital.

- Collapsing and unconsciousness.

Common triggers:

According to the Anaphylaxis Campaign, the most common food triggers of anaphylaxis are:

- Peanuts.
- Tree nuts.
- Sesame seeds.
- Seafood.
- Dairy products.
- Eggs.

Non-food triggers include:

- Wasp or bee stings.
- Natural latex.
- Penicillin and other drugs.

Some people also react after exercise, with or without any other trigger.

See chapter 8 for more information on the symptoms and treatment of anaphylaxis.

Multiple allergies

Some children only ever have one allergy to one specific trigger. But increasing numbers of children are suffering from more than one allergy at a time. This can cause a combination of the main allergic diseases. For example, if your child has hayfever, they may also develop asthma triggered by pollen. Children who have an egg allergy are often prone to eczema and are also at an increased risk of peanut allergy. House dust mite allergy can trigger perennial rhinitis, asthma and eczema.

'Children who suffer from more than one allergic condition may need to see several different doctors, e.g. an allergy specialist, a skin specialist and/or an asthma specialist, to keep their symptoms under control.'

Children who suffer from more than one allergic condition may need to see several different doctors, e.g. an allergy specialist, a skin specialist and/or an asthma specialist, to keep their symptoms under control.

Allergies usually develop in particular stages during childhood, although they often overlap. This progression of allergic disorders is known as the Allergic March. As you can see from the diagram below, eczema is usually diagnosed first in very young babies. This is often followed by food allergies in the first three years of life. As children get older, they become more likely to develop rhinitis and then asthma. However, if your baby has eczema, it doesn't mean that they will go on to develop the other allergies, but it does increase the chances of this happening.

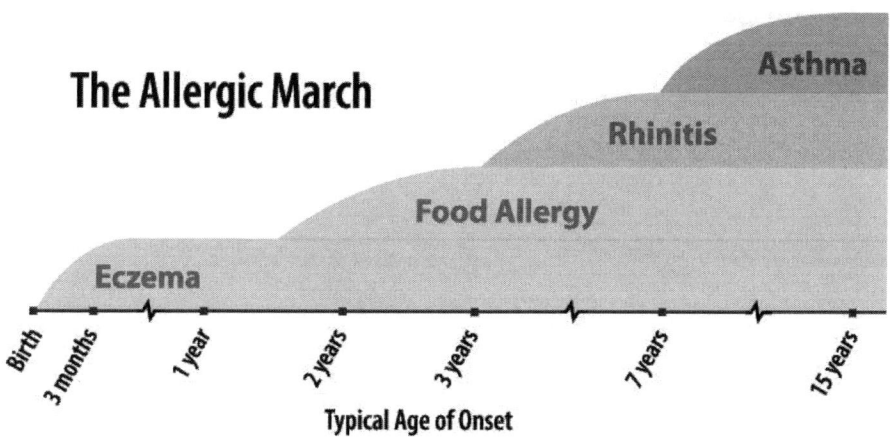

Source: The Immune Tolerance Network.

Growing out of allergies

All parents want to know whether their child will grow out of their allergies. Unfortunately, no one can provide a definite answer. However, an allergy expert should be able to tell you what your child's chances are of being allergy-free as they get older.

- Three-quarters of children grow out of atopic eczema by puberty, according to the National Eczema Society.
- Two-thirds of children will have fewer asthma symptoms as they reach their teenage years, according to Asthma UK.
- Some children do grow out of their food allergies, especially egg or milk allergy, by the age of three years, but around 80% of children with peanut allergy will have the allergy for life.

Summing Up

- Your child may have only one allergy symptom or several symptoms.
- Not all allergy symptoms are easy to identify as they can be similar to other childhood conditions or infections.
- The main atopic diseases are: allergic rhinitis, atopic eczema, allergic asthma, urticaria, oral allergy syndrome, food allergies and anaphylaxis.
- Some children suffer from more than one atopic disease.
- Allergy symptoms can change over time.
- Some, but not all, children will grow out of their allergies.

Chapter Four
Getting a Diagnosis

You should seek medical advice if your child develops any signs of an allergic reaction so that they can receive the most appropriate treatment. Even if their symptoms are very mild or you think you know what they are allergic to, it's important to get a proper diagnosis. This is because some allergies get worse over time or you may find that your child is also allergic to other things that you didn't know about. If your child has eczema or asthma, insist on allergy testing to check whether or not an allergy could be triggering their symptoms.

Be prepared

It isn't always easy to pinpoint allergy triggers, so it helps if you do some research before you consult a healthcare professional. Your child's medical history will help to decide whether or not allergy tests could be helpful, so make sure you provide as many details as possible.

Essential questions

A healthcare professional is likely to ask you the following questions to help identify the specific allergens triggering your child's symptoms:

- How long has your child had the symptoms?
- What were the symptoms?
- How severe were they?
- Has your child had these symptoms before?
- Can you think of anything that may have triggered them, e.g. a new food or high pollen count?

'It isn't always easy to pinpoint allergy triggers, so it helps if you do some research before you consult a healthcare professional.'

- Do the symptoms happen at a particular time of day or in a particular environment, i.e. home or school?
- Do they occur all year round or just at certain times?
- Did you give your child any treatment when the symptoms occurred; if so, what did you give them and what happened?
- Is there a family history of allergies, eczema, hayfever or asthma?

Keep a diary

Make a note of the following each time your child develops the symptoms:

- What your child has recently eaten, touched or breathed.
- Where you were at the time.
- What time of day it was.
- What form the symptoms took.

Research your family history

Allergies tend to run in families, so if you, your partner or your other children have any allergies, write them down, including the triggers and symptoms. Ask any grandparents too, as you may not remember that you had an allergy or eczema as a very young child or how severe it was.

Who to approach

A pharmacist or GP is likely to be your first port of call. The healthcare professional you choose may depend on your child's symptoms and their severity.

> 'A pharmacist or GP is likely to be your first port of call. The healthcare professional you choose may depend on your child's symptoms and their severity.'

Your local pharmacist

Increasing numbers of pharmacists are receiving allergy training through Allergy UK's Accredited Pharmacy Allergy Screening Service. As the service isn't available on the NHS, you will have to pay for the pharmacy consultation and a finger-prick blood test for the most common allergens. The test involves taking a small drop of blood from your child's finger with a sterile single-use lancet (needle), and the results are available in around 30 minutes. Once you have the test results, the pharmacist may give you advice on avoiding the allergens or suggest that you consult your child's GP.

You can find your nearest accredited pharmacist through Allergy UK's website. Look for two valid certificates on display in the pharmacy to prove that the pharmacist has completed the full training.

Your GP

Your GP can deal with most common allergies by providing appropriate medicines and advice. If your child has a severe allergic reaction or non-specific symptoms, such as a rash or wheezing, you should consult your GP straightaway.

Specialist help

Your GP may decide that your child will benefit from being referred to a specialist NHS allergy clinic. The reasons for this include:

- Your child's allergy triggers are unclear.
- Your child has several allergy triggers.
- Your child's allergies are getting worse.
- Simple medicines aren't helping your child's symptoms.
- Your child may be at risk of a potentially serious allergic reaction.

Allergy clinics

Your child should be seen by an allergy consultant who specialises in treating children, called a paediatric allergist, rather than a general allergist. There are very few specialist NHS allergy clinics in the UK, and even fewer paediatric allergists, so you may have to travel to your nearest clinic. The waiting lists can be long, sometimes several months. The British Society for Allergy and Clinical Immunology (BSACI) website provides a list of NHS allergy clinics; see www.bsaci.org.

Your child may also need to be seen by other specialist doctors. For example, if your child has eczema, you may need to see a dermatologist, a doctor who specialises in skin problems.

Your first appointment

- At the initial appointment the allergy consultant will take down a detailed clinical history.
- Your child will be able to have allergy tests performed by specialist staff.
- After the consultation you should be given a comprehensive management plan, including guidance on allergen avoidance, treatment and any training on administering emergency medicines.
- You may need to make a follow-up appointment to discuss the test results or to see if your child's symptoms improve or worsen over time.

Choosing private health

With long waiting lists for NHS allergy clinics, many people choose to see an allergy consultant privately. As with the NHS, there aren't many private consultants specialising in paediatric allergy. Many of the private consultants work in the NHS as well, so your GP should be able to refer you to a suitable consultant.

> 'At one point we were seeing so many different specialists for Jessie's asthma, eczema and allergies that we couldn't keep track of all the appointments. She had to take a lot of time off school and I had to keep finding childcare for the other children. Now we see one paediatrician who sends us to the other specialists only when necessary.'
>
> Gail Flaum, whose six-year-old daughter has eczema and multiple allergies (including egg, nut, chocolate and dust).

If you have private medical insurance, check what your child will be covered for. An initial consultation can cost over £100 and this probably won't include any allergy tests which can cost several hundred pounds.

Allergy testing

Many allergies can be diagnosed from a clinical history alone without the need for allergy tests. However, accurate testing can put your mind at rest and confirm any specific triggers. This may be necessary if your child has a severe allergy or if there is some confusion about whether the symptoms are actually due to an allergy.

Your child shouldn't take any medicines containing antihistamines for a specific length of time before the tests (your GP and allergy consultant will advise you), as these can affect the test results. This includes not only antihistamine syrups but some cough medicines too.

There are many allergy tests available but only two of them are routinely recommended by healthcare professionals:

- Skin prick tests.
- RAST (radioallergosorbent) IgE blood tests.

It's important that the tests are performed by trained doctors or nurses who know how to interpret the results, as the results are meaningless on their own. Home testing allergy kits (using RAST technology) can be as accurate as hospital tests. However, you shouldn't use them without proper medical advice.

'There are only two validated allergy tests; the skin prick test and specific-IgE blood tests.'

Dr George Du Toit, consultant in paediatric allergy at St Thomas' Hospital.

Skin prick test

What is it?

This is the most commonly used allergy test. It tests for up to 25 allergens at a time, with the allergens selected according to your child's medical history. The test is usually performed on your child's forearm, or back if your child has bad eczema.

What it involves:

A drop containing diluted foods or substances is placed on your child's skin and the area is labelled with a marker pen so that the nurse knows what the test liquid contains. The skin beneath the liquid is then gently scratched with a tip of a small needle. This allows the test liquid to enter the skin. If a red, raised, itchy lump, called a weal, develops where the liquid was scratched in, this suggests that your child is allergic to this particular substance. The average weal is 5-10mm in diameter.

The nurse will also use a positive control containing histamine (which everyone should react to) and a negative control containing sterile salt water (which no one should react to). If your child reacts to the negative control, this suggests that their skin is extremely sensitive and the test results may not be reliable.

> 'Test results should always be interpreted by an experienced person who has taken a proper history from the patient.'
>
> John Collard, clinical director at Allergy UK.

Pros:

It's quick, cheap, usually painless and suitable for all ages. You get the results within 15 to 20 minutes. The presence of a weal doesn't tell you how severe the reaction is but shows whether your child reacts to that particular substance. Severe reactions are rare.

Cons:

The test can make your child's arm very itchy for up to 30 minutes. Keep reminding your child not to scratch, as this will affect the results, and distract them with books or toys. It may help if they wear a long-sleeved top that covers their arms.

Blood tests

What is it?

RAST blood tests measure the amount of IgE antibodies in your child's bloodstream. Each IgE antibody is produced to a specific allergen, so your GP or allergy consultant may ask for 'IgE to egg' or 'IgE to peanut'.

What it involves:

You need to take your child for a blood sample at a hospital or GP surgery. The blood sample will be taken from your child's arm and then sent to a central laboratory. The results are usually reported as Classes, where 1 is low and 6 is extremely high. You won't get the results for up to two weeks. In the meantime, your child will need to carry on avoiding any potential allergens as discussed with your GP or allergy consultant.

Pros:

A blood test is useful in children who:

- Are at risk of a severe allergic reaction.
- Have widespread eczema that makes skin prick testing impractical.
- Can't stop their allergy medication safely.

Cons:

- The test isn't popular with children. It's important to reassure your child that the test doesn't last very long, although it can be a little painful.
- The nurse can use some local anaesthetic cream before the test to temporarily numb your child's skin.
- The test is reliable only in eight out of 10 cases and can give false negatives and false positives.
- Although the test shows how much specific IgE antibody there is in your child's blood, it doesn't show how severe your child's symptoms are. For example, a child with high levels of specific antibodies to peanut has a high risk of an allergic reaction, but the reaction itself could be mild or severe.

Other recognised tests

- Skin patch tests investigate delayed allergic reactions, e.g. to foods in severe eczema. They involve sticking metal discs containing the suspected allergen to your child's back for 48 hours. You then return to the clinic so that the doctor or nurse can examine your child's skin for signs of a positive reaction.

- Food challenge tests check your child's response to increasing amounts of specific foods if skin and blood tests don't provide clear results or if your child may have grown out of an allergy. The tests need to be performed in a specialist clinic or hospital in case your child has a severe reaction.
- Lung function tests can check to see if your child has asthma. They involve blowing into a special tube attached to a computer. The tests are usually suitable for children over six years, as young children may find the technique too difficult.

Controversial tests

IgG antibodies are produced by the body in response to various foods but their role in food allergy and intolerance is unclear. There has been some research into the effectiveness of IgG blood tests for food intolerance. However, these tests are not reliable as IgG antibodies to foods are often found in healthy non-allergic people. The only approved test for food intolerance is the elimination diet – see chapter 6.

Vega testing, hair analysis and applied kinesiology are not backed by any clinical research.

Summing Up

- If your child has any allergy symptoms, you should seek medical advice from a pharmacist or GP.
- Your child's clinical history, e.g. symptoms or environment, may provide the key to establishing the allergic triggers, so keep a diary of your child's symptoms.
- Your GP may refer your child to a specialist allergist at an NHS or private allergy clinic.
- Allergy tests can confirm allergy triggers but should be performed by an experienced healthcare professional.
- The most common allergy tests are skin prick testing and RAST blood tests.

'Allergy tests can confirm allergy triggers but should be performed by an experienced healthcare professional.'

Chapter Five

Avoiding Common Allergens

Once you know what your child is allergic to, the next step is to limit their exposure to their allergy triggers. This should reduce their chances of developing the symptoms. However, you'll need to take a sensible approach, getting advice from your child's allergy consultant or GP.

If your child has a food allergy, you'll need to avoid all contact with the culprit foods (see chapter 6). The same goes for latex allergy and drug allergies. But if your child is allergic to airborne allergens, e.g. pollen or house dust mites, it's virtually impossible to achieve complete avoidance and you shouldn't turn your home into a sterile environment.

If you find that some of the avoidance measures aren't working, especially in relation to house dust mites, then there may be no point in continuing with all of them. Even if you do follow the allergy prevention steps in this chapter, it doesn't necessarily mean that your child's symptoms will completely disappear.

'If your child has a food allergy, you'll need to avoid all contact with the culprit foods (see chapter 6). The same goes for latex allergy and drug allergies.'

House dust mites

House dust mites are tiny insects that thrive in warm, humid conditions, especially centrally heated homes. The mites are particularly common in beds, carpets, soft furnishings and even your child's cuddly toys, in fact, anywhere that collects dust.

Your child isn't actually allergic to the mites themselves but to the mites' droppings. The allergy can trigger flare-ups of rhinitis, asthma and eczema, especially in the autumn and winter months when house dust mites are at their highest levels due to central heating.

Take action

- Replace your carpets with a hard flooring that doesn't have any cracks or grooves for dust to collect.
- Dust your surfaces regularly with a slightly damp cloth as this will stop the dust becoming airborne. Don't forget to wipe your child's toys too.
- Buy your child a high bed instead of one near the carpet.
- Use a wooden slatted bed with a big gap underneath for vacuuming.
- Vacuum regularly, every day if possible. Asthma UK suggests using a vacuum cleaner with good suction and a filtered exhaust that doesn't scatter dust. Look for products with high efficiency particulate air (HEPA) filters.
- Use zip-up anti-allergy barrier coverings on bedding, pillows, duvets, mattresses and cushions.
- Wash your child's bedding regularly. Asthma UK recommends a hot wash (at 60°C) once a week.
- Don't keep cuddly toys on your child's bed. Asthma UK suggests that parents put soft toys into a bag in the freezer for a minimum of six hours every one to two weeks to kill house dust mites. Alternatively, you can wash the toys at 60°C.
- Avoid dust traps like cushions and dried flowers.
- Air your house every day to keep it cool and dry. Use a dehumidifier to dry out the air, as this makes it more difficult for house dust mites to survive.
- Clean your soft furnishings with anti-house dust mite chemicals. Professional dust mite removal systems advertise their services through the Yellow Pages, although they may be quite expensive.

'Dust your surfaces regularly with a slightly damp cloth as this will stop the dust becoming airborne. Don't forget to wipe your child's toys too.'

Pollen

According to the National Pollen and Aerobiology Unit (NPARU), grass pollen affects about 95% of all hayfever sufferers and birch tree pollen affects about 20%. Oak tree, plane tree and nettle pollens are also common hayfever triggers.

Different pollens are higher at certain times of the year. If you know which pollen your child is allergic to, see the calendar on the NPARU website to check when your child is most likely to be affected. Some people are allergic to more than one type of pollen, so they suffer from symptoms over a longer period.

Hayfever tends to be worse in built-up areas because air pollution alters pollen so that it is more likely to trigger an allergic reaction.

Take action

- Don't stop your child playing outside – it's healthy for children to have fresh air. However, don't let them out when the pollen counts are high. Check the pollen forecasts on the TV, in newspapers or on the Internet. Pollen levels tend to be highest in the early morning (7-10am) and late afternoon (4-7pm).
- Grow insect-pollinated plants (usually with brightly coloured flowers) in your garden and replace your lawn with paving.
- As soon as your child comes indoors, give them a shower and wash their hair and clothes.
- Give your child some wraparound sunglasses to wear as these will stop pollen flying into their eyes. Look for British Standard BSEN 1836:1997 to ensure the sunglasses offer a safe level of ultraviolet (UV) protection.
- Keep your doors and windows closed. Mow the lawn when your child isn't at home and don't let your child play outside for the rest of the day.
- Keep your car windows closed. Some cars can be fitted with pollen filters.
- Avoid drying clothes outside.

'When the pollen count is very high, we don't let Samuel play in the garden or go to a park for too long.'

Vicki Gilbert, whose eight-year-old son, Samuel, has hayfever.

- Brush or wash your cat or dog when they come indoors as they can carry pollen in their fur.
- Smear petroleum jelly inside and under your child's nose to trap pollen. This can also soothe any sore skin caused by a constant runny nose.
- If your child likes playing sports, avoid grassy areas and play on hard surfaces or Astroturf instead.

Pets and other animals

Cats are more likely to trigger allergies than any other animal, closely followed by dogs. The main cat allergen (Fel d1) is usually found in the cat's saliva. When cats lick themselves, they spread the allergen onto their fur and skin. It can then be passed through the air onto furnishings, people's hands and clothing.

Horses, rabbits, guinea pigs and birds are also common allergy triggers. Animal allergies can cause a range of symptoms.

Take action

- Try to find a new home for your pet. If you can't, or don't want to, make sure that you keep them out of the key living areas, especially the bedrooms.
- Always make sure your child washes their hands after stroking any animals, even the family pet.
- Bathe cats and dogs at least once a month.
- If friends or family have pets, you could ask them to vacuum and dust extra carefully before you visit and to keep the pet out of the room that day.

Moulds and fungi

Moulds and other fungi release tiny seeds called spores which can trigger asthma attacks, allergic rhinitis, wheezing or itchy eyes. They are found indoors and outdoors – anywhere that is damp and warm, including compost heaps, farms, leaves, grass and poorly ventilated rooms, such as kitchens and bathrooms. They can be a particular problem in the late summer and autumn, especially in the evenings.

Take action

- Keep your house well ventilated; open the windows regularly and keep the bathroom and kitchen doors closed.
- Make sure your clothes are completely dry before putting them away.
- Look out for any mould growth or musty smells in your house.
- If you find any damp patches on your walls, treat them as soon as they appear. Look in the Yellow Pages for a local damp treatment company.
- Don't let your child walk through compost heaps or wet leaves as these may contain mould spores.

Medicines

Drug allergies are more common in adults than in children. Antibiotics, especially penicillin and its relatives, are the most common drug allergy triggers, and even very small amounts can trigger a reaction. Some other medicines (e.g. ibuprofen) can trigger asthma attacks, although these are not true allergic reactions. This is why people who have asthma are often advised to avoid these medicines. Your child can also be allergic to other ingredients in medicines rather than the medicines themselves.

'Antibiotics, especially penicillin and its relatives, are the most common drug allergy triggers, and even very small amounts can trigger a reaction.'

Take action

- Make sure your child always wears medical ID jewellery so doctors don't give that particular medicine to your child, especially in an emergency.
- Make sure your child's allergy is stated clearly on all their medical notes – doctor, dentist, etc.
- Always tell a pharmacist which medicines and ingredients your child

is allergic to before you buy any product over the counter or obtain a prescription medicine. Penicillin-related antibiotics tend to have names ending in 'cillin'.

Insect bites and stings

In the UK, most insect-related allergic reactions are to wasps and bees. The allergy is triggered by enzymes in the insect venom/poison. Bees and wasps have different enzymes, so your child is likely to be allergic to one but not the other. Some people are allergic to bites from mosquitoes, midges, gnats and fleas.

Most insect bites and stings cause redness and swelling at the site of the injury, even in non-allergic people. This is a normal response and isn't usually dangerous. In people who are allergic to insect bites and stings, the reaction is much more severe and immediate. The symptoms can range from a rash to life-threatening anaphylaxis, e.g. severe swelling, vomiting, faintness, wheezing and breathing problems.

> 'If a wasp or bee comes near your child, don't try to swat it away, however tempting it may be. Insects are more likely to sting if they are upset or disturbed, so try to remain as calm and still as possible.'

Take action

- Grow more wind-pollinated plants (usually with small, green-yellow flowers) in your garden and don't leave flowers on the table, indoors or outdoors.
- Don't use fragranced products on your child or let them wear bright colours or flowery prints.
- Don't leave opened sugary or sweetened foods and drinks outside because these attract insects.
- A good-quality insect repellent will repel biting insects, but it won't work against wasps or bees.
- If a wasp or bee comes near your child, don't try to swat it away, however tempting it may be. Insects are more likely to sting if they are upset or disturbed, so try to remain as calm and still as possible.

- Don't let your child walk outside barefoot, especially on grass, as bees tend to fly close to the ground.
- Keep rubbish bins covered and don't leave any windows open.
- Avoid picnic areas and clover fields.

Latex

Latex, a gluey plant sap, makes natural rubber more elastic. It's found in many rubber-based products, including balloons, rubber gloves, household goods, sports equipment, clothing and medical devices. Anyone can develop an allergy to latex, but the allergy is becoming more common in children who have repeat surgical procedures or hospital stays, e.g. those with spina bifida, and are therefore exposed repeatedly to latex-containing hospital equipment (e.g. gloves, adhesive plasters and dressings, catheters, etc).

Your child doesn't need to come into direct contact with latex to experience a reaction. Some latex gloves used in hospitals are coated with powder to make them easier to take on and off. When they are taken off, the powder is released, spreading tiny particles of latex into the air.

'Latex is found widely in the environment and in day-to-day products. Avoidance can be very difficult.'

John Collard, clinical director at Allergy UK.

Take action

- The only way to avoid a reaction is to avoid latex-containing products, including latex or rubber dummies and baby bottle teats, stretchy rubber toys, balloons, rubber bands, some adhesive tapes and bandages, some shower curtains and some clothing elastic.
- Make sure your child wears ID jewellery at all times, in case they need emergency medical treatment.
- Your child's medical records must have a note on the front to state that they have latex allergy.
- Contact the Latex Allergy Support Group for more information. See help list for details.

Summing Up

- Once your child has been diagnosed with an allergy, you should try to limit their exposure to any known triggers.

- If your child is allergic to house dust mites, you won't be able to cut out dust completely. However, you should clean and dust your home thoroughly and regularly. You may wish to make some changes to your flooring and furnishings.

- If your child is allergic to pollen or insects, you will need to take precautions when they are outdoors.

- If your child is allergic to specific medicines or latex, this should be stated clearly on their medical records.

Chapter Six

Coping with Food Allergies

Food allergies affect around one in 17 children in the UK and cases are rising fast. This is why I have devoted a whole chapter of the book to food allergies.

If your child has a food allergy, the only way to keep them safe is to avoid any foods to which they are allergic. However, if your child has an allergy to common foods, e.g. milk, or multiple food allergies, this can be more of a challenge.

Is it really an allergy?

The only reliable way to know for certain if your child has a food allergy is to get them professionally diagnosed (see chapter 4). It's important not to self-diagnose the allergy as you may be putting them at risk of nutritional deficiencies, e.g. a lack of calcium if you cut out dairy products.

Is it a food intolerance?

According to the British Dietetic Association (BDA), around 5-8% of children have a food intolerance rather than an allergy. The symptoms aren't usually life-threatening, but they can cause significant discomfort and distress. They include diarrhoea, weight loss, bloating and allergy-like rashes. There's no reliable test for most food intolerances, except coeliac disease (gluten intolerance), other than the elimination diet (see later on in chapter).

> 'According to the British Dietetic Association (BDA), around 5-8% of children have a food intolerance rather than an allergy.'

Allergy versus intolerance symptoms

Food allergies	Food intolerance
Usually immediate reaction.	Slower or delayed reaction.
Small amount of substance triggers symptoms.	Can usually tolerate small amounts of substance; excessive or prolonged exposure usually triggers symptoms.
Often severe symptoms.	Much milder symptoms.
Same reaction each time.	Reaction may vary.

Is it a reaction to food additives?

Some children have an asthma attack or develop a rash on exposure to certain food additives, usually sulphites, benzoates and tartrazine.

There's also evidence that some artificial food colourings can affect children's behaviour, making them seem hyperactive. This is a form of food intolerance rather than an allergy. Common culprits are:

- Sunset yellow (E110).
- Quinoline yellow (E104).
- Carmoisine (E122).
- Allura red (E129).
- Tartrazine (E102).
- Ponceau 4R (E124).

Contact the Hyperactive Children's Support Group (HACSG) to learn more about the link between food and children's behaviour. See help list for contact details.

Get some dietary advice

Everyone should eat a healthy balanced diet, but this isn't always straightforward if you have a food allergy or intolerance. You won't want to restrict your child's diet so much that they begin to resent eating or worry about whether foods are safe. This is why you should seek professional dietary advice from a dietitian. A dietitian can advise on healthy eating for allergic or intolerant children and suggest suitable food substitutes, especially for wheat or dairy.

Most people see a registered dietitian on the NHS after a referral by their GP or allergy consultant. However, you can also arrange to visit a dietitian privately. Registered dietitians are regulated and governed by an ethical code set by the BDA. You can find a dietitian through the BDA's website (see help list).

Elimination diets

A dietitian may suggest that your child tries an elimination diet to check for food intolerances. It involves removing specific foods or ingredients from your child's diet to see if the symptoms clear up. You then reintroduce these foods, one at a time, to see if the symptoms recur.

An elimination diet is a long process and can be very stressful, which is why it needs to be supervised by a registered dietitian or doctor. It doesn't work for everyone and isn't suitable for anyone with a true food allergy.

Avoiding food allergens

Food allergens can turn up in places you would least expect, even in toiletries and other products. It can be very confusing at first but you will gradually learn what your child can and can't eat or use.

The following lists overleaf are not exhaustive – there may be other ingredients you should look for as well, which is why it's vital that you get advice from a registered dietitian. The Anaphylaxis Campaign can also provide further information (see help list).

'Advice from a specialist dietitian, particularly in older children, enhances the child's confidence by providing better coping strategies, especially when eating out.'

Professor Gideon Lack, Head of Children's Allergy Service, Guy's and St Thomas' NHS Foundation Trust and Professor of Paediatric Allergy, King's College London.

Peanuts and tree nuts

- Tree nuts include almonds, hazelnuts, walnuts, cashews, Brazil nuts and pecans.
- Peanuts are also listed as arachis oil, groundnuts, earth nuts, peanut oil and monkey nuts.
- Most allergy specialists recommend that a peanut-allergic child avoids tree nuts, and vice versa, but speak to your allergy consultant about this.
- Check the ingredients of cakes, biscuits, ice cream, desserts, chocolate bars, cereal, cereal bars, vegetarian foods (e.g. veggie burgers), salads and salad dressings.
- Avoid marzipan (almond) and praline (hazelnut) confectionery and Chinese, Thai and Indonesian cooking.
- Nut oils, especially almond, may be found in some toiletries.
- Peanuts aren't actually nuts, they are legumes. So your child may also be allergic to other legumes like lentils, chickpeas and peas. Your allergy consultant should test your child for a reaction.

'Some manufacturers do pay to have a nut-free factory, but most of them don't and several products may be made on the same production line or factory floor.'

Sesame seeds

- Foods containing sesame include hummus, halva and tahini, vegetarian foods, biscuits, health food snacks and Chinese and Japanese products.
- Avoid Chinese meals as these may contain sesame oil.
- Sesame is also used in breads, so bakery products may be contaminated.

Egg

- Look for albumin, binder, coagulant and emulsifier on the label. Lecithin is often derived from egg rather than soya.
- Egg can be hidden in many foods and even shampoo and cosmetics.
- Some egg-allergic children can eat well-cooked egg (e.g. in cake) without any symptoms.

- The MMR vaccine (and the single measles jab) can contain trace amounts of egg protein. According to the Paediatric Allergy Group of the BSACI, there's no evidence that the MMR vaccine is a problem for children with egg allergy. Allergy UK recommends that all egg-allergic children should still receive the MMR jab to protect them against measles, mumps and rubella. When your child has the vaccine, make sure you keep their medicines close by in case they have a reaction. If your child has experienced anaphylactic reactions in the past, the vaccine may be given in hospital.

Cow's milk

- Cow's milk can be found not only in dairy products but also in a range of foods, including muesli, sausages and packet soups.
- Look for casein, whey, sodium caseinate and calcium caseinate in the ingredient list.
- Children may react to milk in toiletries (e.g. soaps) on their skin.
- Some children can cope with trace amounts in cooked foods, e.g. cake.

Seafood

- Check pasta sauces, stocks, table sauces (Worcester sauce contains anchovies), soups and Oriental foods.
- Children's vitamin and mineral supplements may contain fish oils.
- If your child reacts to one type of fish or shellfish, you may need to avoid all fish or shellfish as cross-contamination is very common.

Wheat

- Most common foods contain wheat. These include bread, pasta, bran, semolina, wheat-based breakfast cereals, pizza, biscuits, cakes and even soy sauce and gravies. However, wheat-free alternatives are often available.

> 'We don't have any peanuts in the house and don't eat them if we go out (even without the children), just in case we bring crumbs home. The grandparents' homes are also peanut-free.'
>
> Vicki Gilbert, whose six-year-old son, Adam, has peanut allergy.

> 'When Jessie was first diagnosed, it was scary to shop for food. There are so many different ingredients in everything and many of the descriptions aren't obvious. Now I can break down the ingredients in my head, but I still find it hard to get information about all the different food additives.'
>
> Gail Flaum, whose six-year-old daughter has eczema and multiple allergies (including egg, nut, chocolate and dust).

- Gluten is a protein found in wheat, as well as barley and rye. If your child is allergic or intolerant to wheat, don't give them gluten-free foods. 'Gluten-free' foods are not the same as 'wheat-free' foods. These may still contain some other wheat proteins, making them unsuitable for people with wheat allergy or intolerance.

Shopping guide

The first time you go shopping after your child is diagnosed can be very bewildering. The easiest foods to buy are raw ingredients or unprocessed foods, such as fresh fruit and vegetables. However, you still need to be vigilant.

Follow these tips for stress-free shopping:

- Allow yourself plenty of time to check the labels. Don't shop in a hurry because this is when you are most likely to make a mistake.
- Make a list of all the foods, and brands, you know your child can eat and stick with them.
- If you're not sure, don't buy it. Contact the manufacturer or retailer directly for a list of ingredients.
- Remember that ingredients can change, so always check the labels even if your child has eaten that product before.
- If you are buying unwrapped food, e.g. from a deli counter, check that there's no cross-contamination.
- Bakery goods, especially bread, can be a problem for nut allergy sufferers as you can't guarantee that there's no contamination from cakes or biscuits.
- Remember to look at toiletries and cosmetics. Some bath products may contain traces of milk, egg, nuts or even fruits.
- You can sign up for free allergy alerts from the Food Standards Agency, Allergy UK and Alert4allergy (see help list for details).

'Free from' foods

- Most supermarkets and health food stores have a 'free from' range. You can request a 'free from' list from them to help you find safe alternatives to things your child can't eat. This will cover most common allergies. Ask for updates because manufacturers change ingredients from time to time.
- Search on the Internet for allergy-free food companies, such as Kinnerton chocolate (nut-free), Alpro (milk and dairy alternatives) and Trufree (wheat-free and gluten-free).

Reading food labels

Since November 2005, all pre-packaged food is required by EU law to be labelled with 14 allergenic ingredients, even if they are present in trace amounts. These are:

- Cow's milk.
- Eggs.
- Shellfish.
- Fish.
- Soya.
- Peanuts.
- Tree nuts.
- Wheat.
- Sesame.
- Mustard.
- Celery.
- Sulphites.
- Molluscs.
- Lupin.

Allergy information on food labels should make shopping easier, but it can still be very confusing. For example, the words 'may contain traces of' do not tell you whether the product actually contains that particular allergen. This may be because the manufacturer can't guarantee that the product is completely allergen-free, as there's always a chance that a piece of food, e.g. a nut, could have been lodged in a machine without anyone realising. Some manufacturers do pay to have a nut-free factory, but most of them don't and several products may be made on the same production line or factory floor.

In reality, there's always a risk of contamination, even with pre-packaged foods. The safest option is to avoid any products that say 'may contain' or 'may contain traces of'. But only you can make this decision on behalf of your child.

Adapting your home

Turning your house into a safe zone isn't necessarily the best, or most practical, solution. However, this will depend on what your child is allergic to, how allergic they are and how important the foods are in the family diet.

- Peanuts should be quite easy to keep out of the home as they aren't an essential snack. If your child is very allergic, they may react to peanut on your breath or skin – if this is the case, all household members need to avoid peanuts, even when they are out of the house.

- It's more difficult to keep very common foods, such as milk or wheat, out of the home completely. However, you may need to if your child experiences severe reactions. Otherwise, you will need to teach your child that certain foods are out of bounds and keep these foods well out of reach.

- Cross-contamination can occur, especially in the kitchen, as food can get trapped in tiled surfaces or inside ovens. Keep your surfaces scrupulously clean and sweep up after meals.

Cooking meals

Let your child join in with family meals as much as possible so they don't feel like they are missing out. If your child has multiple allergies, it's usually easiest to cook all of their meals from scratch.

- If you need to cook special foods for your child, cook large batches and freeze them.
- Plan your weekly menu in advance, with a different meal each day, preferably over a two-weekly or monthly cycle. This will make sure that your child doesn't get bored.
- Learn to experiment. You may need to adapt recipes to suit your child's needs, e.g. substitute soya cream for dairy cream.
- You can buy special diet cookbooks from health food stores, bookshops, pharmacies, websites and allergy associations. The Vegan Society has recipes for egg-free and dairy-free foods (see help list for details).

Summing Up

- Don't diagnose your child's food allergy yourself.
- Consult a registered dietitian to make sure your child continues to eat a healthy, varied diet.
- Allergens can be hidden in many foods, so read the labels carefully.
- 'Free from' foods are available from supermarkets and health food stores – these may be useful for dairy and wheat allergies.
- Let your child join in with family meals as much as possible.

Chapter Seven

Allergy Treatments

This chapter looks at the most common allergy medicines that your child may be prescribed. This isn't a complete list, as there are many different treatments available. Many allergy medicines are used for more than one allergic condition. Some prevent allergy symptoms from occurring, while others treat them when they arise.

Allergy medicines are available to buy from pharmacies. However, it's important to get a prescription from your GP for your child's medicines, as this will ensure that you are giving your child the correct dose. Some over-the-counter medicines shouldn't be given to children without advice from a GP.

It's natural to worry about side effects, particularly when it comes to children. But most side effects are very rare, especially if you use the medicines as directed.

Some allergy medicines contain corticosteroids. Many people worry when they hear the word 'steroid', but these steroids are not the same as those used by bodybuilders and athletes. Your GP or pharmacist will be able to reassure you that children are usually given a very low dose of steroid which is less likely to cause any side effects.

Remember that the medicines are only a small part of the whole management process, so make sure your child avoids their allergy triggers (see chapter 5) and uses self-help measures where possible to ease their symptoms.

Management plans

Your GP or allergy consultant should write out a management plan for your child so you know exactly how to use the medicines and what to do when the symptoms flare up.

The treatment needs to be reviewed at regular intervals. This is because your child may need a larger dose or different medicines as they get older or their symptoms may change over time. Some medicines shouldn't be taken for long periods because this can increase the risk of side effects.

Specific allergy medicines

Antihistamines

How they work: antihistamines block the action of histamine to reduce allergy symptoms. They work best if you take them before an allergic reaction occurs, although they can be taken during a reaction to stop further histamine release. They are suitable for most allergies, including rhinitis, urticaria and insect bites/stings. If your child has hayfever, an antihistamine can relieve sneezing and a runny nose, but it's less effective for a blocked nose.

> 'Allergies do change over time, so every allergy patient should be reviewed regularly.'
>
> John Collard, clinical director at Allergy UK.

How to use them: antihistamines can be prescribed in various forms.

- Sugar-free elixirs and syrups. Promethazine, an older-type antihistamine, is fast-acting, so it's used for acute allergy symptoms, e.g. itching or a rash. However, its effects last only for a few hours. Newer-type antihistamines (e.g. cetirizine, loratadine) can be taken once a day to prevent or treat hayfever or perennial rhinitis.

- Creams or ointments. These are usually used for the treatment of non-allergic reactions to insect bites and stings.

- Eye drops/nasal spray. These are applied directly to the eyes or nose.

Safety:

- Older-type antihistamines can cause drowsiness, headaches, dizziness, a dry mouth and blurred vision if they are used regularly.

- Newer-type antihistamines are less likely to cause these side effects.

Adrenaline

How it works: this natural hormone is used for anaphylactic shock and other allergic emergencies. It relaxes muscles in the lungs to aid breathing, tightens the blood vessels to increase blood pressure, reduces swelling of the face or lips and stimulates the heart.

How to use it: adrenaline is fast-acting but should be given as soon as the symptoms occur. Auto-injectors (pre-assembled syringes fitted with a needle) are simple to operate in emergencies – even children can learn to use them. They are usually prescribed in batches of two, as some reactions may require a second dose.

Safety: see chapter 8 for more details on using adrenaline safely.

Steroid nasal sprays

How they work: steroid nasal sprays contain very low doses of corticosteroids which dampen down the immune system. They reduce symptoms from airborne allergens, such as house dust mites and pollen.

How to use them: you need to use the sprays every day. They can take several days to work.

Safety:

- The sprays may make the nose and throat dry or uncomfortable.
- They are unlikely to cause side effects when used for short periods.
- Your child's height will need to be monitored if they use the sprays regularly for longer periods.

Cromoglicate-type drugs

How they work: these are used in nasal sprays and eye drops for rhinitis. They are thought to work by blocking the immune system cells that release histamine.

How to use them: the drugs take several weeks to work, so you need to start taking them every day well before the hayfever season.

'Samuel starts taking his hayfever medicines well before the pollen season, usually from the end of March. He uses an antihistamine syrup, steroid nasal spray and sodium cromoglicate eye drops. If we forget to use them every day, his symptoms flare up.'

Vicki Gilbert, whose eight-year-old son, Samuel, has hayfever.

Safety:

- Side effects are uncommon.
- There may be some initial stinging or burning when putting in the eye drops and some irritation from the nasal spray.

Eczema treatments

These include emollients and topical steroids.

Emollients

How they work: emollients provide a protective oily barrier on the surface of the skin. They moisturise the skin and reduce itching. Some also contain antibacterial agents, but these should be avoided unless your child has an infection or is prone to them.

How to use them: emollients need to be used regularly whether the skin is dry or not. They can be used in various forms:

- Creams, lotions and ointments. These are applied directly to the skin.
- Bath and shower oils. These are added to a bath or used in the shower.
- Soap substitutes. These are an effective alternative to soap.

Safety:

- Don't use aqueous cream (a soap substitute) as a leave-on emollient because it can cause irritation.
- Some emollients can trigger a skin reaction, so try new products on a small patch of skin first.
- Leave 30 to 60 minutes between applying an emollient and applying a topical steroid or topical calcineurin inhibitor (see overleaf).
- Bath products can make the skin slippery, so be extra careful when holding your child.

> 'Emollients are often underused. Children with severe eczema may need emollients four to five times a day.'
>
> Margaret Cox, chief executive of the National Eczema Society.

Topical steroids

How they work: topical steroid creams, ointments, lotions and gels treat eczema flare-ups by reducing inflammation. Some are combined with an antibiotic to fight infections.

How to use them: steroid preparations should be used in small doses as soon as a flare-up occurs. Your GP will show you how much to apply.

Safety:

- Topical steroids are safe if you use them as directed.
- They can thin the skin if they are used for long periods in high doses. However, children are usually prescribed the milder strengths in small doses which are unlikely to cause side effects.

Wet wrapping

Wet wrapping involves using layers of damp bandages over liberal amounts of emollients. This improves the absorption of emollients and keeps inflamed skin cool, reduces itching and prevents scratching. Wet wrapping must be used under medical supervision.

Safety:

- Wet wrapping shouldn't be used on infected skin as it can make it worse.
- Wet wrapping can increase the risk of folliculitis (a bacterial infection of the hair follicles) which may need to be treated with antibiotics.
- It is time-consuming and can be uncomfortable for the child, so you need to be shown how to use the wraps properly by an experienced healthcare professional.
- Sometimes wet wrapping is used with topical steroids, but this can increase the risk of side effects, so your child will need to be monitored carefully.

> 'Topical steroids are safe if they are used appropriately; using them is better than having terrible eczema.'
>
> Margaret Cox, chief executive of the National Eczema Society.

Calcineurin inhibitors

How they work: these relatively new treatments (tacrolimus ointment and pimecrolimus cream) are applied to the skin to reduce inflammation and itching. They may be used in children over two years when topical steroids don't work or aren't suitable.

Safety:

- There's no risk of skin thinning.
- Doctors don't yet know enough about their long term safety.

Asthma treatments

There are two main types of asthma medicines: relievers (usually blue or grey) and preventers (usually brown, red, orange or white). Your child will be shown how to use them by a doctor or asthma nurse. Children under five years may need to use a large-volume spacer device which makes an inhaler easier to use. A spacer has a mouthpiece at one end and a hole for the inhaler in the other. If your child can't use the mouthpiece, they will probably need a face mask as well.

Reliever inhalers (beta agonists)

How they work: they are breathed in through the mouth to open up the airways.

How to use them: use them when asthma symptoms, e.g. wheezing or coughing, occur. Their effects last for three to six hours.

Safety:

- These are very safe, with few side effects. Your child can't overdose on them.

Preventer inhalers (inhaled steroids)

How they work: these are breathed in through the mouth straight into the airways. These are usually prescribed for asthma if your child needs a reliever more than twice a week or if their symptoms disturb their sleep more than once a week.

> 'There are two main types of asthma medicines: relievers and preventers. Your child will be shown how to use them by a doctor or asthma nurse.'

How to use them: your child will be prescribed the lowest dose possible to control their symptoms. Preventers need to be used regularly, even when your child has no symptoms.

Safety:

- Side effects are rare as the steroids go straight to your child's airways and very little is absorbed into their body.
- In large doses, over a long period of time, steroids can slow down growth, so your child's height will need to be monitored.
- Steroid treatment can lower your child's resistance to chickenpox.
- There's a small risk of a sore throat or tongue and a hoarse voice. Asthma UK suggests rinsing out your child's mouth and brushing their teeth after using a preventer inhaler.

Other medicines

Steroid tablets

- Your child may be prescribed a short course of steroids after a particularly severe asthma attack or allergic reaction.
- Steroid tablets can cause mood swings and increased hunger.
- Your child's growth may need to be monitored.
- Your child will need to avoid contact with chickenpox or measles for three months after taking steroids, as these infections could be more serious than normal.

Antibiotics

- These kill bacteria, so they can be used to reduce the risk of, or treat, infections.
- They may be given for a flare-up of eczema or a chest infection in a child with asthma.

'Asthma UK suggests rinsing out your child's mouth and brushing their teeth after using a preventer inhaler.'

- They can be given as tablets, syrup or cream.

Leukotriene receptor antagonists

- These block leukotrienes (inflammatory chemicals produced during an allergic reaction).
- They are an alternative to steroid treatments as they have fewer side effects.
- They may be effective in atopic eczema, asthma, perennial rhinitis or urticaria.

Anti-IgE drugs

- These stop IgE antibodies from binding to mast cells and triggering a reaction.
- In the UK, they are licensed for the treatment of severe and persistent allergic asthma in the over-12s.

Immunotherapy

- Immunotherapy alters the immune system so that it no longer reacts to allergens.
- It may be given to children who react to airborne allergens, such as pollen or house dust mites, when they haven't responded well to anti-allergy drugs.
- Your child will usually be given an injection or a tablet or spray under their tongue (sublingual immunotherapy) containing the allergen to which they are sensitised.
- They will be given gradually increasing amounts of the allergen until they no longer react to it.
- For most allergies, immunotherapy is only available from specialist centres because it can sometimes cause potentially serious allergic reactions. A sublingual tablet is now available on the NHS for children over five years with severe grass pollen allergy.

- The treatment isn't suitable for children under five years.

Medicine management

- If your child needs to carry medicines with them for emergencies, keep the medicines together in one bag. For examples of what to keep in your child's medicine bag, see chapter 8.
- Keep the medicine bag by the front door but out of your child's reach, or in your handbag, so that you don't forget it when you leave the house.
- If your child needs medicines at particular times of the day, leave notes in prominent places, such as by your child's bed, or set an alarm to remind you.
- Use the medicines as directed by your child's GP. If you have any questions, e.g. about the dose or side effects, ask your GP or a pharmacist.
- Even if you see some improvement, don't stop using the medicines as this could make your child's symptoms return.
- Your child might be prescribed other medicines or need vaccinations or over-the-counter products. Always tell your GP or pharmacist what other medicines your child has been prescribed to avoid drug interactions, even if they are used only occasionally.

Summing Up

- Children need a range of different medicines to control allergies.
- The main allergy medicines are antihistamines, adrenaline, steroid nasal sprays and cromoglicate drugs.
- Emollients and topical steroids are the main eczema treatments.
- Children with asthma usually need inhaled beta-agonists, possibly with a daily inhaled steroid.

Chapter Eight

Dealing with Medical Emergencies

No matter how much you try to keep your child safe by avoiding all their known allergy triggers, there's always a risk that a medical emergency will occur. It can be frightening when your child has an asthma attack or anaphylactic reaction, especially the first time. It's therefore important that you, your child and anyone who looks after your child are able to deal with severe allergy or asthma symptoms and know how to use the treatments properly.

Emergencies can happen when you're away from home, so make sure you keep a mobile phone with you at all times. If you are planning a day trip, or even visiting friends, check in advance where the local hospital is and, if possible, obtain the phone number of the nearest doctor.

Your child's medicine bag

Make sure your child's medicine bag is clearly labelled, can be securely fastened and is easy to recognise so that everyone knows that it contains your child's medicines. You can buy children's bags specifically designed for carrying medicines. Don't use the bag for anything else, as it can easily become cluttered. You don't want your child rifling through the bag looking for a toy or colouring pencils and leaving their medicines behind.

The bag should contain details of your child's symptoms, treatments and allergy triggers. On the next page are some examples of what you may wish to keep in your child's medicine bag, depending on what medicines they need to carry, what they are allergic to and the size of the bag.

'Jessie's medicines don't fit in a small enough bag for her to carry. But I don't want to give her too much responsibility yet anyway as she is only young. I keep the medicines in a toiletries bag in my handbag so I know we always have them with us. We also have medicines at the grandparents' houses and at school.'

Gail Flaum, whose six-year-old daughter has eczema and multiple allergies (including egg, nut, chocolate and dust).

Examples of items you might like to include:

- Your child's allergy medicines (e.g. antihistamine, adrenaline autoinjector, asthma inhalers or emollient creams).
- Management plan from your child's GP or allergy consultant.
- Symptom checklist to help people identify an emergency.
- Clear instructions on what to do in an emergency.
- Medicine instructions and diagrams, e.g. patient information leaflets.
- Details of what your child is allergic to.
- A list of suitable foods for when they stay with friends or family or go to parties (food allergies only).
- A suitable food item for your child (food allergies only).
- Your emergency contact phone numbers in case your child isn't with you when the emergency occurs.
- GP's contact details.
- MedicAlert details if your child is a member; see chapter 10.

> 'Adam wears a small blue hip bag, which is instantly recognisable. It's big enough for a bottle of antihistamine, two EpiPens, his management plan and our emergency contact details.'
>
> Vicki Gilbert, whose six-year-old son, Adam, has peanut allergy.

Treating asthma attacks

According to Asthma UK, a child is admitted to hospital in the UK every 16 minutes because of their asthma. Asthma attacks are more likely to occur if your child's asthma is not kept under control or if they have been previously admitted to hospital for an asthma attack. An asthma attack can be triggered by your child's usual allergy triggers, a viral infection, like a cold, or exercise. Even mild asthma can worsen suddenly and require emergency treatment.

To keep your child's asthma under control, follow your child's personal asthma plan which will have been devised in discussion with your GP. This means avoiding your child's known asthma triggers, using the medicines as directed by your GP and monitoring your child's symptoms carefully.

If your child's symptoms are worsening, don't ignore them as this will mean that an asthma attack is more likely to occur. Make an urgent appointment with your GP or asthma nurse so that the medicine can be adjusted to bring your child's asthma back under control.

Symptom check

During an asthma attack, the muscles in the airways tighten up so your child finds it more and more difficult to breathe. Some attacks are worse than others; a very severe asthma attack can make the airways close so much that not enough oxygen reaches the vital organs such as the heart and lungs, resulting in a medical emergency. It's important to treat all asthma attacks, however mild, before they reach this stage.

According to Asthma UK, signs that your child is having an asthma attack include:

- Your child's reliever doesn't help their symptoms.
- Your child's symptoms (cough, breathlessness, wheeze or tight chest) are getting worse.
- Your child is too breathless to speak, eat or sleep.

Asthma UK treatment guidelines

Asthma UK suggests that you follow these steps during an asthma attack:

- Give your child their reliever inhaler (usually blue) immediately.
- Sit your child down and ensure that any tight clothing is loosened. Don't let them lie down.
- If there's no immediate improvement during an attack, continue giving your child one puff of the reliever inhaler every minute for five minutes or until their symptoms improve.
- If your child's symptoms don't improve in five minutes, or you are in doubt, call 999 or a doctor urgently.
- Continue to give them one puff of the reliever inhaler every minute until help arrives.

- Keep your child calm and reassure them, as stress will exacerbate the situation.

Hospital treatment

The hospital treatment will depend on your child's age and the severity of their symptoms.

Not all asthma attacks need hospital treatment. But if your child's symptoms are not eased by their reliever inhaler or are getting worse, you need to be seen by a doctor straightaway. The doctor will send your child to the Accident & Emergency (A&E) department at the hospital if the attack continues. If your child's symptoms are severe, you may prefer to go straight to the hospital. If your child is admitted to hospital, make sure you have details of their regular medicines with you.

'If your child's symptoms are worsening, don't ignore them as this could mean that an asthma attack is more likely to occur.'

- Your child may be given oxygen and higher doses of inhaled reliever medicines (salbutamol or terbutaline) via a nebuliser. A nebuliser is a machine that creates a fine mist of medicine which is then breathed into the lungs through a mask or mouthpiece.
- Your child may also need other medicines like intravenous salbutamol, steroid tablets (prednisolone) and/or inhaled ipratropium bromide.
- Antibiotics are not usually necessary because most asthma is worsened by viral infections rather than bacterial infections.

For more information, see the 'British Guideline on the Management of Asthma', produced by the British Thoracic Society and the Scottish Intercollegiate Guidelines Network in May 2008.

After a severe attack

Make an appointment with your GP or asthma nurse for an asthma review within 48 hours of your child's attack.

- Your child's inhaler technique should be checked.
- If your child only uses reliever inhalers, they may need a preventer inhaler as well.

- Your child's personal asthma plan may need to be revised.
- You will need another review with your GP within one to two weeks after the asthma attack to make sure your child's symptoms are being controlled more effectively.
- Your child may be referred to a paediatric asthma clinic.

Asthma attack cards

Asthma UK can supply you with a credit-card sized guide on what to do during an asthma attack. English and Welsh versions are available from Asthma UK's website or Asthma UK's Support and Information team. See help list for details.

Treating anaphylactic reactions

In January 2008, the UK Resuscitation Council reported an increase in the rate of hospital admissions for anaphylactic reactions. Anaphylaxis is a frightening experience and can occur within a couple of minutes of allergy symptoms appearing. However, death from anaphylaxis is very rare and most children with food allergies don't experience severe symptoms.

If your child is prescribed adrenaline, you or your child should carry it with you at all times, even if all previous reactions have been mild. No environment can be completely safe. Children can react to a new allergen at any time, or may even react to something they have previously tolerated. Also, you can't predict how much allergen your child will be exposed to or what the reaction will be.

> 'Anaphylaxis is a frightening experience and can occur within a couple of minutes of allergy symptoms appearing. However, death from anaphylaxis is very rare.'

Symptom check

An anaphylactic reaction can affect your child's whole body. According to the Anaphylaxis Campaign, possible symptoms include:

- Alterations in heart rate.
- Swelling of the throat and mouth.
- Abdominal pain, nausea and vomiting.

- Difficulty breathing or swallowing.
- Weakness or floppiness, due to a drop in blood pressure.
- Steady deterioration.
- Collapse or unconsciousness.

Not everyone will necessarily experience all of these symptoms.

Treatment plan

You, your child and all carers need to know how to recognise an anaphylactic reaction and when and how to administer life-saving adrenaline. Your GP or allergy consultant will devise an emergency treatment plan that includes when you should use an adrenaline auto-injector. The directions will vary from child to child.

- As soon as your child has a mild allergic reaction, e.g. itching or rash, your GP or allergy consultant may suggest that they take a dose of antihistamine, usually chlorphenamine liquid. However, this antihistamine doesn't treat anaphylaxis.
- If your child experiences any of the symptoms associated with anaphylaxis (see earlier), they need adrenaline immediately. You should use the adrenaline auto-injector prescribed by your GP or allergy consultant. This is why it is so important to keep your child's allergy medicines with them at all times. If you have not been prescribed adrenaline (usually because your GP or allergy consultant did not think that your child was at risk of anaphylaxis), consult a doctor or go to the hospital immediately.
- Your child's symptoms should improve straightaway. If not, use a second adrenaline auto-injector after five to 10 minutes.
- Call 999 for an ambulance. All children should be taken to hospital after being given adrenaline, even if their symptoms have improved.

Using adrenaline auto-injectors

Pre-loaded adrenaline auto-injectors (Anapen or EpiPen) are available on prescription only.

- Each auto-injector pen contains one adrenaline injection for emergency use.
- Your child will be prescribed either the adult version or the junior version, depending on their bodyweight. Junior versions are suitable for children weighing 15 to 30kg (2 stone 5lb to 4 stone 9lb).
- You need to inject the auto-injector into your child's thigh. It can be used through clothing.
- It's important to read the instructions carefully as the Anapen and EpiPen are activated in slightly different ways. The EpiPen should be jabbed into the thigh after pressing down the firing button, while the Anapen needs to be held against the thigh before pressing the firing button.
- The auto-injectors need to be held against the thigh for 10 seconds to allow the adrenaline to enter the muscle. The area of injection should then be lightly massaged for 10 seconds.
- Not all of the auto-injector's contents are discharged when you use it. However, the auto-injector can't be used again and should be discarded safely after use.
- The auto-injectors have a safety cap to prevent accidental firing and can be used with one touch. They are light, compact and portable.

Safety guidelines

The storage instructions will vary according to the manufacturer, so read the patient information leaflet carefully. The general advice is:

- Don't use adrenaline after its expiry date – get auto-injectors with the latest expiry date you can from the pharmacy (usually around 12 months).
- Seek immediate medical advice in the event of an accidental injection,

as this may result in a rise in blood pressure that needs to be monitored. Accidental injections into the fingers or thumb may stop the blood flow to the affected area.

- Side effects can include rapid heart rate, breathing problems, paleness, irregular or fast heartbeat, sweating, nausea, tremors (shaking) and headache.

- Adrenaline is sensitive to light and air, so keep it in its outer carton. Don't store it above 25°C or refrigerate or freeze it.

- Don't use an auto-injector device if the solution becomes coloured or contains visible particles. When exposed to air or light, adrenaline will become pink or brown.

- Adrenaline should be injected into the outer thigh, not the buttocks.

Training devices and expiry service

You can obtain free auto-injector training pens from the Anapen and EpiPen suppliers or your GP/allergy consultant so that you, your child and all carers can practise using the device.

ALK-Abello also provides a free EpiPen Expiry Alert Service which reminds you by letter, email or SMS text message when your EpiPen needs to be replaced. This service is available to EpiPen and EpiPen Junior users. Anapens are distributed by Lincoln Medical Ltd. EpiPens are manufactured by ALK-Abello Ltd.

The following EpiPen and Anapen diagrams have been reproduced with the kind permission of ALK-Abello Ltd and Lincoln Medical Ltd respectively.

How to use your *Anapen*®
Adrenaline (Epinephrine)

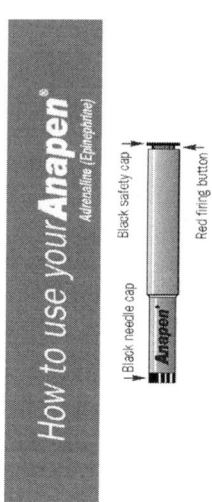

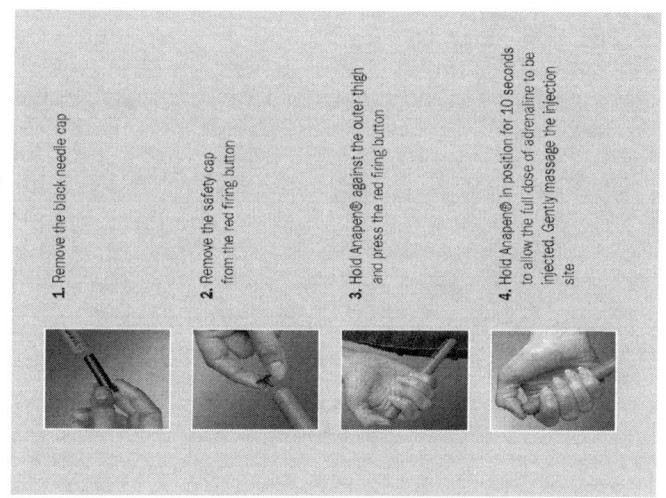

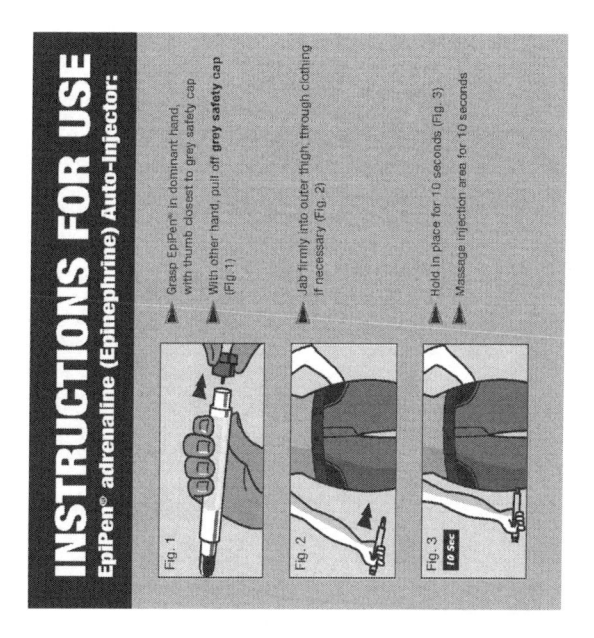

- Black needle cap
- Black safety cap
- Red firing button

1. Remove the black needle cap
2. Remove the safety cap from the red firing button
3. Hold Anapen® against the outer thigh and press the red firing button
4. Hold Anapen® in position for 10 seconds to allow the full dose of adrenaline to be injected. Gently massage the injection site

INSTRUCTIONS FOR USE
EpiPen® adrenaline (Epinephrine) Auto-injector:

- Grasp EpiPen® in dominant hand, with thumb closest to grey safety cap
- With other hand, pull off **grey safety cap** (Fig. 1)
- Jab firmly into outer thigh, through clothing if necessary (Fig. 2)
- Hold in place for 10 seconds (Fig. 3)
- Massage injection area for 10 seconds

'You can obtain free auto-injector training pens from the Anapen and EpiPen suppliers or your GP/allergy consultant so that you, your child and all carers can practise using the device.'

Summing Up

- Emergencies like an asthma attack or anaphylactic reaction can occur at any time, so it's important to be prepared.
- Carry your child's medicines with you at all times in a designated recognisable bag.
- Your GP will write out an allergy or asthma treatment plan, including what you should do in an emergency.
- If your child has an adrenaline auto-injector, make sure you know how to use it and follow the safety guidelines.

Chapter Nine

Using Complementary Therapies

According to the Prince's Foundation for Integrated Health, research shows that 10% of people in the UK use complementary therapies every year, and 46% are expected to use complementary therapies during their lifetime. People use complementary therapies for various reasons; they may be dissatisfied with conventional treatments or they may think that a holistic or natural approach is safer, even though this isn't always the case.

Most people with allergies who use complementary therapies tend to have one of the main allergic diseases – asthma, atopic eczema or rhinitis. This chapter focuses on the main therapies that you may want your child to try.

The therapies can't cure long term medical conditions and can't be used to treat emergency situations like an asthma attack or anaphylactic reaction. The therapies won't provide a quick-fix solution as you usually need to use them over a long period of time before you see any benefits. With some therapies, such as homeopathy, the symptoms often get worse before they get better. However, sometimes they may help to make the symptoms more bearable so that your child relies less on conventional medicines.

If you decide to try a complementary approach, it's important that you speak to your child's GP or allergy consultant and other healthcare professionals first. Some therapies may interact with your child's treatment, while others aren't suitable in certain medical conditions, including asthma or allergies. You shouldn't consult a complementary practitioner until your child's allergy has been properly diagnosed, or stop your child's conventional medicines unless your GP advises it.

'The therapies can't cure long term medical conditions and can't be used to treat emergency situations like an asthma attack or anaphylactic reaction. However, sometimes they may help to make the symptoms more bearable so that your child relies less on conventional medicines.'

Complementary therapies can be expensive, so make sure you explore all the options first. There's limited research available, although there is a lot of anecdotal evidence. A lack of clinical research doesn't necessarily mean that a therapy doesn't work, but it does mean that it needs more reliable research studies before doctors are prepared to recommend it.

Finding a practitioner

It's important to find a reputable practitioner who isn't only used to treating children, but also has experience in dealing with your child's particular allergy.

'It's important to find a reputable practitioner who is not only used to treating children, but also has experience in dealing with your child's particular allergy.'

Recommendation is best, so ask around to see if anyone you know has consulted a local practitioner for the same condition. Your GP may also be able to refer you. Ideally, you should consult a medically qualified practitioner, e.g. a GP or pharmacist who has completed further training in complementary therapies.

Not all doctors are willing to prescribe complementary medicines, often because of a lack of resources. The types of treatment you can access will depend largely on where you live. There are five NHS homeopathic hospitals in the UK: in Bristol, Glasgow, Liverpool, London and Tunbridge Wells. If your GP won't refer you to a practitioner, you will have to pay for the treatment yourself. Some levels of private medical insurance cover complementary therapies, so check your policy if you have one.

Ask the right questions

If you are referred to a complementary practitioner, or choose to contact one privately, it's important to make sure that they are fully qualified and are an accredited member of the appropriate professional organisation.

You should ask the practitioner the following questions:

- Do you belong to a recognised professional organisation with a code of practice?
- What are your qualifications and for how long did you train?
- Can you tell me more about your professional experience?

- Is your complementary approach suitable for children?
- Do you have professional indemnity insurance in place?
- Are your records confidential?
- Do you take a full medical history?
- Will you speak to my child's GP or other healthcare professionals if necessary?
- How many treatments is my child likely to need, and what is the likely cost involved?
- What does the treatment usually involve?
- What are the potential side effects or risks?
- Will it interfere with any conventional treatments?
- Are you on the register of my private medical insurance company?

Acupuncture

Acupuncture involves inserting very fine needles at key points into the body. For children, some acupuncturists use massage or pressure rather than needles, but this will depend on your child's age.

Acupuncture is used mainly for painful conditions, such as migraines and backache. Some people also use it for asthma and rhinitis, but there is limited research. According to Asthma UK, acupuncture may be effective for people whose asthma is triggered by an allergy, but less effective for those whose asthma is exercise-induced.

Acupuncture is generally safe, with few side effects or complications. However, make sure that the acupuncturist is fully qualified and uses single-use disposable acupuncture needles. Avoid acupuncture if your child is allergic to any metals, as the needles could trigger a reaction.

Further information is available from the British Acupuncture Council (which represents professional acupuncturists in the UK) and the British Medical Acupuncture Society (BMAS), whose members are healthcare professionals, i.e. GPs.

> 'Acupuncture is used mainly for painful conditions, such as migraines and backache. Some people also use it for asthma and rhinitis, but there is limited research.'

Aromatherapy

Aromatherapy uses essential oils extracted from flowers, plant roots, bark, leaves, etc. The essential oils may be inhaled, added to the bath or applied to the skin in creams or during a massage. There's no evidence that aromatherapy can help allergies or asthma, although it can be used for relaxation and stress-related conditions. Some essential oils, such as tea tree oil, have been proven to have antibacterial and antifungal properties.

Essential oils are highly toxic and shouldn't be applied neat to the skin, especially in children. They must be diluted in a carrier oil first, although even diluted oils can irritate the skin. Some carrier oils are derived from nuts such as almond, so it's important to tell the aromatherapist if your child has a nut allergy.

Further information is available from the Aromatherapy Council, the governing body for the UK aromatherapy profession, and the International Federation of Professional Aromatherapists which maintains a register of practising members. See help list for details.

The Buteyko method

The Buteyko method was first developed in the 1950s by a Russian doctor called Konstantin Buteyko. It involves learning specific breathing exercises. A Buteyko practitioner will show your child how to do the breathing exercises and may advise you on other ways to manage your child's condition, such as dietary changes.

Research in 2002, funded by Asthma UK, found that Buteyko breathing may help to reduce asthma symptoms and the use of reliever inhalers, but not necessarily improve the underlying condition. According to the 'British Guideline on the Management of Asthma', produced by the British Thoracic Society and the Scottish Intercollegiate Guidelines Network in May 2008, the Buteyko method should be considered to help patients control asthma symptoms.

Further information is available from the Buteyko Breathing Association (see help list for details).

> 'According to the "British Guideline on the Management of Asthma", produced by the British Thoracic Society and the Scottish Intercollegiate Guidelines Network in May 2008, the Buteyko method should be considered to help patients control asthma symptoms.'

Chinese herbal medicine

Some medical research suggests that traditional Chinese herbs may be effective in the treatment of atopic eczema. One clinical trial in August 2007, published in the *British Journal of Dermatology*, found that a formulation of five Chinese herbs ('pentaherb concoction') was more effective than placebo (dummy) pills in improving the quality of life and reducing the need for topical steroids in children with moderate to severe atopic eczema.

Chinese herbs must be prescribed by a properly trained practitioner. However, there have been reports of adverse reactions. For example, some products are poor quality, some have contained harmful ingredients, such as steroids, and others have been contaminated with heavy metals.

Further information is available from the Register of Chinese Herbal Medicine which regulates the practice of Chinese herbal medicine in the UK. See help list for details.

Homeopathy

Homeopathy is based on the principle of 'like cures like'. This means that a remedy that is used to treat particular symptoms in an ill person will produce the same symptoms when it's given to a healthy person. The remedies are derived from mineral, plant and animal sources and contain highly diluted substances. Homeopaths believe that the more dilute the remedy is, the more effective it will be. When treating a patient, homeopaths take into account a range of physical, emotional and lifestyle factors.

Homeopathic remedies are often used to relieve allergy symptoms or to reduce the immune response to allergens – called desensitisation. It's a popular therapy for children as it's very gentle and has no side effects. Some research has found that hayfever, perennial rhinitis and asthma respond well to homeopathy, but doctors say there isn't enough evidence yet to recommend the therapy as a treatment.

Further information is available from the British Homeopathic Association which promotes homeopathy practised by doctors and other healthcare professionals (e.g. pharmacists), and the Society of Homeopaths which can provide a register of trained homeopaths. See help list for details.

Medical herbalism

Medical herbalism uses extracts from the roots, leaves, flowers and stems of various plants. There's growing medical evidence that some herbs can help in allergic conditions, e.g. butterbur in hayfever and evening primrose oil in eczema.

Some herbal remedies are available over the counter from pharmacies, health food stores and supermarkets. These are very generalised remedies, so you should take your child to a qualified medical herbalist for an individualised approach. Herbs can also interact with conventional medicines and may even cause side effects themselves, which is why you shouldn't self-treat.

Further information is available from the National Institute of Medical Herbalists. See help list for details.

Nutritional therapy

Nutritional therapy involves the use of dietary and nutritional advice, food supplements and special diets, as well as the avoidance of toxins. Some practitioners offer sound medical advice, but others make dubious claims. You can also buy natural dietary products or supplements from pharmacies and health food stores, but many of them aren't backed by research.

A nutritional therapist isn't the same as a dietitian. If your child has a food allergy or is following a restricted diet, it's important that you consult a registered dietitian instead. There's not enough evidence to suggest that extra nutrients can prevent or treat allergy, asthma or eczema symptoms. According to Asthma UK, there's no evidence that children who already have asthma but don't have food allergies will benefit from any special diets or food supplements.

> 'A nutritional therapist isn't the same as a dietitian. If your child has a food allergy or is following a restricted diet, it's important that you consult a registered dietitian instead.'

Some nutritional products can trigger allergies or may not be suitable for people with certain medical conditions or taking some medicines. For example, Royal Jelly and propolis should be avoided by people with asthma and allergies, as they may cause serious side effects.

You can search the British Association for Applied Nutrition and Nutritional Therapy's (BANT) website for a local practitioner. The Nutritional Therapy Council's website can confirm whether a practitioner is registered if you know their name. See help list for details.

Summing Up

- Complementary therapies can't cure long term medical conditions or treat emergency reactions, but they may be able to make some symptoms more bearable.

- There is very little reliable medical research to show that complementary therapies can effectively treat allergies, asthma or eczema.

- Your GP may be able to refer you to a local practitioner. However, you will usually have to pay for the treatment yourself.

- Speak to the practitioner to make sure that you feel comfortable before you use them. In particular, check their professional insurance, qualifications and treatment approach.

- Don't change your child's medical treatment or stop their usual medicines without seeking advice from your GP first.

Chapter Ten

Raising a Confident Child

According to the Anaphylaxis Campaign, just as you teach your child about other dangers in life, such as road safety or not to touch a hot oven, it's important that you teach them about their allergy from an early age. You will want them to learn how to recognise and treat their symptoms so that they can manage their own allergy by the time they go to secondary school.

Deal with your emotions first

When your child is first diagnosed, you may feel a whole host of emotions: worry, despair, anxiety, fear, etc. It's natural to feel like this, especially if the allergy could be life-threatening, as you're taking on a huge responsibility.

Some parents blame themselves or experience feelings of denial. But you could be putting your child's life at risk if you don't tackle the allergy head on by learning more about it and building good habits.

Your child won't become independent if you aren't comfortable in dealing with their allergies yourself, as children pick up on their parents' insecurities. The more confident you are, the more confident your child will be as they grow up.

> 'When your child is first diagnosed, you may feel a whole host of emotions: worry, despair, anxiety, fear, etc. It's natural to feel like this.'

Get some support

When you first tell your friends and family, you may get various reactions. Some may offer helpful advice and support, some may be too uncomfortable to discuss the issue, while others may not understand the severity of the allergy and will think you are over-reacting. If you find that your close friends or family aren't supportive, it's easy to feel isolated. But remember that you're not alone – healthcare professionals, national charities and local support groups can also provide essential support and advice.

Often one parent spends more time as the main carer, but it's important that the other parent isn't excluded. Communication is the key – talk about your feelings, discuss day-to-day management issues and make decisions together. Think of your other children's needs too – they may feel that they're not getting enough attention. Give them their own one-to-one time and make sure they don't miss out on activities because their allergic sibling can't take part.

It can be very tiring if you're juggling work, other children and/or household responsibilities with looking after an allergic child, so ask for help from family or friends if you need anything like extra childcare or shopping. Make sure everyone knows that all help, however small, is appreciated so that they offer again!

Give yourself a break from time to time. For example, book a babysitter so that you can go to the shops or have an evening out. Or just lock the bathroom door and immerse yourself in a warm bath once the children are in bed.

Discuss allergies with your child

It's vital that even very young children understand what an allergy is, so speak to them about their symptoms and treatment from an early age. Choose your words carefully according to your child's age and maturity so that they aren't frightened unnecessarily. You will find that you can go into more detail as your child gets older.

The Anaphylaxis Campaign warns that you should be careful of the language you use when you talk about the dangers. Although it's important that your child is aware of the seriousness of the allergy, it won't help if you make constant references to death. On the other hand, if your child thinks that their allergy just makes them feel a little under the weather, rather than causing severe symptoms, they may be more likely to take risks.

Be patient with your child – it may take them a while to get used to their allergy. For example, children with a food allergy may tell you that lots of foods are making their mouth 'tickly' when they are first diagnosed, even foods they aren't allergic to. Take each episode seriously and get used to these false alarms. Eventually your child will feel more comfortable about the food they eat.

> 'Children should be aware of what they need to avoid and why. But they shouldn't be wrapped in cotton wool or be denied access to events and activities unnecessarily.'
>
> John Collard, clinical director at Allergy UK.

Some children with allergies grow up feeling different to their peers. Explain that lots of children have medical conditions, e.g. diabetes, and that they aren't alone. You shouldn't hide the fact that your child has an allergy – the more people who know about it, the safer your child will be. Make sure your child has people to talk to so they can also get some support if they need it.

Tips on teaching primary school children

- Young children quickly learn to tell others which foods/allergens they need to avoid, so make sure they know exactly what they are allergic to.
- Teach your child how to recognise their allergens. Keep a scrapbook of pictures and words associated with their allergy, e.g. wasps and bees, different nuts, so that they know what to look for. If they have a food allergy, don't just show them pictures of the raw ingredients they should avoid; cut out pictures or labels of different branded products as well and show them the foods on the supermarket shelves.
- Use rewards or positive reinforcement, e.g. kisses and cuddles, every time your child recognises an allergen, remembers to ask questions, etc. If your child makes mistakes, don't dwell on it or embarrass them in front of other people.
- Role play can help your child learn to deal with tricky situations, e.g. being offered food at parties, shopping or sharing with friends.
- Buy a toy doctor or nurse set so that your child can familiarise themselves with equipment like stethoscopes or syringes.
- Discuss what could happen in an emergency. For example, practise with a trainer auto-injector pen or talk through an asthma attack.
- If your child has a food allergy, use the words for food substitutes wisely to avoid confusion, e.g. soya drinks rather than soya milk.

Tips on dealing with teenagers

- As your child reaches the teenage years, you'll need to strike a balance between encouraging independence and making them overanxious.

'How you discuss eczema with your child will depend on them to some degree. You can accidentally make your child feel different when they are not actually bothered by their eczema.'

Margaret Cox, chief executive of the National Eczema Society.

- Allergic children are often aware of their triggers and know how to steer clear of them. However, older children may feel under pressure to take risks, so it's worth reminding them regularly of the basic rules to follow. Don't nag your child though, as this could have the opposite effect.

- Give your child a more active role in decision-making so that they can take over some of the responsibility. Explain the importance of their medicines and how to use them and discuss how to overcome difficult situations.

- Take your child's needs into account so they feel that you take them seriously. If they grow up feeling that their wishes are important, they will be confident enough to speak up if they need to and will be able to handle peer pressure.

- Gradually give your child more responsibility. For example, if they have dust allergy, encourage them to keep their room clean and show them how to vacuum.

- Teach your child how to read food labels and order food safely at canteens and fast food restaurants. Practise whenever you eat out by letting them order their own meal under your supervision.

- Encourage your child to be open with their friends about their allergies.

- Explain to your child that they are not alone. If you don't know any other teenagers with allergies, look for local support groups through the national charities or your GP surgery.

> 'Maya uses public transport to get to school. She carries her EpiPen with her at all times and wears a MedicAlert bracelet.'
>
> Jo Woolich, whose daughter has nut allergy and started secondary school last year.

Useful resources for parents

- *The Diary of Cyril the Squirrel*, available from the Anaphylaxis Campaign, has been written for children aged three to seven years to learn about nut allergy.

- The *New Kid* video, also available from the Anaphylaxis Campaign, is aimed at children aged five to nine years with a food allergy.

- Asthma UK's Kick Asthma website (www.kickasthma.co.uk) is aimed at children and young people with asthma. Visitors to the website can play games, look up health information and email an asthma nurse specialist for advice.

- The National Eczema Society produces a booklet for teenagers with eczema.

Wearing ID jewellery

Your child should wear medical ID jewellery at all times if they have a severe allergy or are at risk of a severe reaction, just in case you're not there in an emergency. If your child is very unwell, they may not be able to tell someone what their allergy is which could delay the treatment.

Various companies sell medical ID jewellery, e.g. Velcro wristbands or fashionable bracelets, but make sure that the products are child-friendly – i.e. waterproof, washable and durable. Registering your child with the MedicAlert Foundation, a charity that supplies medical ID jewellery, will give you additional peace of mind as healthcare professionals can call a 24-hour emergency telephone number to access the wearer's details anywhere in the world in over 100 languages. Contact details are included in the help list.

Get your child used to wearing the jewellery every day, just like an adult wears a watch, even for swimming or sports. Some children have been known to sleep in the Velcro wristbands, although this can irritate eczema! If an older child or teenager isn't keen on wearing the jewellery, stress that wearing it will give you peace of mind so that they can be more independent.

> 'Be upfront about eczema. If people stare, tell them that it's only eczema, it's not catching, lots of people have it and your child doesn't like being stared at.'
>
> Margaret Cox, chief executive of the National Eczema Society.

Coping with eczema

Applying emollients can be very time consuming, but if you don't do this on a regular basis, this can make eczema flare up. Speak to your healthcare professional about ways to make your child's eczema management routine more bearable.

- The best emollient to use is the one that your child prefers, as they will then be happy to use it frequently.
- Build emollients into your child's daily routine and make it as fun as possible with games, stories, etc.

- Don't worry if you make a mess with emollients at bathtime – this is all part of the fun.
- If your child is very itchy, ask your GP about anti-itch products. The National Eczema Society has a factsheet providing tips on distracting a child with severe itching.

Medicine management

- Your child may need to keep medicines with them at all times, even pots of emollients. Start this habit early on so it becomes second nature, although the level of responsibility you give to your child will depend on their maturity.
- If your child has too many medicines to fit in a small bag, you may have to carry the medicines for them.
- Many teenagers like to hide the fact that they are carrying medicines. Stress that this is nothing to be ashamed of.
- Don't let them carry the medicines loose in their pocket, as they are likely to lose them. There are other discreet ways of carrying medicines, such as in a mobile phone case or camera case, so ask your child what they feel most comfortable with. Girls may be happy to carry around a bag of their choice, but boys may be more reluctant to do this. You can buy plain coloured hip bags or EpiPen cases or tubes from Kidsaware or Yellow Cross.

> 'We keep wet sheets of kitchen towel in the freezer. If Jessie's eczema flares up, we can take out a sheet to put over her skin. The sheets are much more pliable than ice packs.'
>
> Gail Flaum, whose six-year-old daughter has eczema and multiple allergies (including egg, nut, chocolate and dust).

Summing Up

- You need to be confident about managing your child's allergy before you teach your child about their symptoms and treatment.
- Get support from family, friends, healthcare professionals and national charities.
- Choose your words carefully when you discuss allergies with your child.
- Teenagers may feel under pressure to take risks, but explain the importance of managing their allergy properly.
- Your child should wear medical ID jewellery if they have a severe allergy. They should also carry their medicines with them at all times if they need them.

Chapter Eleven

Allergies at School

When your child is a baby or toddler, you or a reliable carer will always be nearby to keep an eye on them. But once your child goes to school or nursery, you'll be handing over this responsibility to someone else who is likely to have several children to look after at the same time.

It's natural to worry about whether your child will be safe when you're not there. What if they eat another child's food? What if no one recognises that they are having an allergic reaction? As your child gets older and goes to secondary school, you're likely to have extra concerns. Your child will have to take more responsibility for their own allergy management and there may not be anyone to monitor them.

Voice your concerns

If you have any worries, discuss them with your child's GP or nurse. You will also need to speak to the head teacher before your child starts a new school or a new school year.

You will need to discuss:

- How your child's allergy symptoms and management could affect their schooling.
- How your child can still be involved with all aspects of school life so that they feel as normal as possible.
- How the school can stop your child coming into contact with their individual allergy triggers.
- How the school may have to be flexible with certain rules, e.g. wearing ID jewellery.

'If you have any worries, discuss them with your child's GP or nurse. You will also need to speak to the head teacher before your child starts a new school or a new school year.'

- How new issues can arise during the school year, e.g. dusty building sites near the school or staff changes.
- How the school can guarantee there will always be a teacher nearby who will be able to recognise an allergic reaction.
- How your child's medicines will be managed.

Remember that it can be a daunting time for your child too, so encourage them to speak to you and their teachers if they are worried about anything or are experiencing problems, such as bullying, from other children.

Check the school policies

It's the school's responsibility to have the necessary procedures in place to deal with allergies, including policies on medicines management and supporting children with medical needs. Staff should attend regular training sessions on administering medicines, especially adrenaline auto-injectors and asthma inhalers. If the school doesn't have the right policies in place, speak to the head teacher.

The Department of Health's report 'Managing Medicines in Schools and Early-Years Settings' (2005) provides advice for schools and their employers. The report provides specific information on asthma, diabetes, epilepsy and anaphylaxis, as well as managing medicines forms for staff to complete. The report can be downloaded from www.teachernet.gov.uk/wholeschool/healthandsafety/medical/.

The Medical Conditions at School Partnership is a group of organisations working together to support schools. School staff can download resources from www.medicalconditionsatschool.org.uk, including a medical conditions policy pack.

Draw up a protocol

As a parent, you are obliged to tell the school about your child's allergy and its treatment. Supplying an up-to-date, individualised management plan, called a 'protocol', will ensure that the school staff understands your child's medical

> 'Samuel doesn't like going anywhere without his sunglasses when the pollen count is high. Although most children aren't allowed to wear sunglasses for school, the teachers know that his eyes will flare up if he doesn't wear them.'
>
> Vicki Gilbert, whose eight-year-old son, Samuel, has hayfever.

needs. The protocol should be written in association with the school, your child's GP and the school nurse. It needs to be updated regularly, especially the emergency contact numbers, and should be reviewed at the beginning of each school year.

According to the Anaphylaxis Campaign, a protocol should include:

- Symptoms.
- Emergency procedure.
- Medication.
- Allergen management.
- Staff training.
- Precautionary measures.
- Professional indemnity.
- Consent and agreement.

You can download sample protocols and other documents from the websites of the following charities: Anaphylaxis Campaign's 'Allergy in Schools', Allergy UK, Allergy UK's Blossom Campaign, Asthma UK and the National Eczema Society. See help list for details.

Pre-schools, nurseries and primary schools

While your child is still young, their teachers or carers will need to have control over their day-to-day allergy management. As your child gets older, you can discuss how they can become more involved, e.g. putting on emollients and recognising foods they need to avoid.

Young children are less able to avoid foods that may harm them, so pre-schools and nurseries will need to take additional steps to keep your child safe. Allergy alert stickers, T-shirts and wristbands can be useful aids to make sure that staff are aware of your child's allergies. Put the stickers on their lunchboxes and schoolbags, as other children may have similar designs.

> 'Many schools have a "no touch" policy, so parents have to go in every break time to put emollients on their child. The sooner your child learns to self-manage, the better.'
>
> Margaret Cox, chief executive of the National Eczema Society.

Your child's medicines

If your child has an adrenaline auto-injector or asthma inhaler, these should be kept in a designated central location in the school.

- Check which staff members are responsible for looking after the medicines and administering them if necessary.
- Make sure your child's teacher has immediate access to the medicines. The medicines shouldn't be locked away.
- Keep all of your child's medicines together in one box with a list of emergency telephone numbers and instructions. Put a photograph of your child on the front so there's no doubt who it belongs to, and your child's name and class. Label each medicine separately and check the expiry dates regularly – if possible, obtain medicines that will last the whole school year.
- Your child's teachers, classroom assistants and lunchtime supervisors must be trained in using the medicines and should have professional indemnity insurance (legal cover).
- If your child has eczema, you will need to keep emollients at school. Make sure the teachers are aware that emollients can be messy and take time to apply. Younger children may not be able to apply the emollients themselves, so their teachers will need to help. Some schools have a 'no touch' policy, so you may have to go into the school to apply the emollients yourself.

> 'The school nurse insisted on speaking to Maya at the beginning of the year and showed her how to use an EpiPen.'
>
> Jo Woolich, whose daughter has nut allergy and started secondary school last year.

Secondary schools

At secondary school your child is likely to have less help from the teachers, but the school nurse may be able to provide some support.

- Most secondary schools are too large to keep medicines in a central location, so your child will need to keep their medicines with them.
- If your child travels to and from school on public transport, they should avoid travelling alone, although this can't always be helped.
- They should keep their medicines handy, wear their ID jewellery and remain vigilant at all times.

Avoiding specific triggers

Whatever your child's age, you will need to think about how their main triggers can be avoided. You will also need to think about after-school clubs and class outings.

During lessons or activities

Discuss with the teachers which lessons are likely to pose a problem. Here are some of the issues that may arise:

- Animal allergies: pets in classrooms, visits to farms or pet centres.
- Allergies to chemicals: soaps, paints, glues, detergents, chalk, sand, clay or craft materials in most lessons but especially art, science or food technology.
- Hayfever: pollen in outdoor PE or class outings.
- Dust: sitting on the floor or dusty carpets.
- Asthma: chalky boards. In PE your child will need to carry an inhaler with them on the sports fields.
- Insect allergy: open windows, any outdoor lessons, break times or activities. Your child may need to wear long sleeves and trousers in the summer.
- Eczema: getting overheated from sitting next to radiators or playing sports, washing hands after art lessons and irritation from uniforms which may be made from wool or synthetic fibres and resin glue. You can buy uniforms made from 100% cotton from www.eczemaclothing.com and www.lint-kids.com.
- Food allergies: cereal packets, egg boxes and other food packaging during craft activities, cookery lessons and food technology.
- Latex allergy: balloons, some modelling materials and even glue on stickers, e.g. on fruit.

During mealtimes

If your child has a food allergy, you will have to decide whether they should have school dinners or packed lunches. This will depend on the catering policy and how prepared staff are to deal with different allergies.

Your school may have a nut-free policy in place. However, some experts believe that this can lead children into a false sense of security and that children should get used to an environment where their triggers could be present at any time.

Speak to the teachers and catering staff about the following issues:

- The school should have a list of children with details of their food allergies, a photograph and their class prominently displayed in the dining hall.
- Ask if your child can be given their meal before the other children to guarantee clean utensils.
- Children make a lot of mess when they eat, so ask if spillages can be cleared up straightaway.
- If your child has school dinners, check the menu in advance. The catering staff should have a list of ingredients available.
- Check the seating arrangements as some schools have a nut-free zone. If your child sits with the same children regularly, ask their parents to stress the importance of not sharing food. If possible, ask if these children can also have lunches free from your child's allergens.
- When other children hand out their birthday treats in the classroom, make sure your child doesn't miss out. You could provide the teacher with a full, labelled treat box for your child and replenish it regularly.

'Your school may have a nut-free policy in place. Some experts believe that this can lead children into a false sense of security.'

On school trips

School trips, especially overnight stays, can provide additional risks.

- If you are worried that the location could aggravate your child's allergies (e.g. a trip to a farm), ask if your child can stay behind.

- Make sure the supervising teacher carries your child's medicines with them and knows how to use them.
- Discuss the food in advance – ask if your child can take their own packed lunch.
- If you are particularly worried, arrange to go on the outing – parental help is usually welcomed!

Coping with school work and exams

- If your child has needed to take extra time off school because of their allergies, e.g. poor sleep or regular doctor's appointments, make sure they catch up on the work they have missed. If they are falling behind, see if they can get some extra help.
- When it comes to exams, make sure your child revises early on so that they don't have to cram. Stress and worry, or a lack of sleep, can make allergy symptoms worse and affect a child's performance.
- Visit your child's GP or nurse at least a month before the exams to discuss their allergy management. Make sure that they have enough medicines to last the exam period.
- Summer exams coincide with the peak pollen season. Children with hayfever must remember to use their medicines regularly and stay indoors when the pollen count is high.
- Your child may need to take their inhaler into the exam room as stress can make asthma worse.
- If your child's hands are painful from eczema, they may be able to use a tape recorder or have extra time to complete the papers. Make sure they have extra emollients with them at school.
- If severe symptoms are affecting your child's performance, their GP may be able to write a certificate asking for their medical condition to be taken into account when the papers are marked.

'Summer exams coincide with the peak pollen season. Children with hayfever must remember to use their medicines regularly and stay indoors when the pollen count is high.'

Summing Up

- Make an appointment with your child's teachers to discuss their allergy management.
- Check the school policies and write a protocol outlining your child's symptoms and treatment.
- Discuss how to avoid allergy triggers in certain lessons.
- Allergy symptoms can affect your child's academic performance, especially during exams.

Chapter Twelve
Living with Allergies

As your child grows up, you'll want to keep them safe, but it's also important that they don't feel different or miss out on activities. You will need to weigh up the pros and cons of every situation or occasion. For example, do you let your child have a fun time at a party or on a day trip but run the risk of a reaction? Or do you say no? Your decision may depend on how well you can predict the severity of the reaction or how easily you will be able to take precautions.

Most serious allergic reactions happen out of the home, so keeping your child's medicines handy should be a matter of routine. Remain vigilant, whatever the activity or situation, especially with young children.

See chapter 5 for tips on avoiding common allergens and chapter 6 for more specific information on food allergies.

Eating out

Restaurants can cater for most food allergies, but eating out can be more difficult if your child has multiple allergies.

- Choose the restaurant carefully, e.g. no Oriental or Indian food if your child is allergic to nuts. Even going out for tea can be a problem as cakes and biscuits may contain eggs, wheat, milk and/or nuts.
- At canteens and self-service counters there may be no one to ask about ingredients. Go at quieter, off-peak times and choose basic foods like a jacket potato.
- Always ask to speak to the manager or chef when you arrive and tell them about your child's allergy so that the food can be kept separate. Warn them about cross-contamination from utensils, spillages, etc.

> 'It's important to put the risks in perspective and to allow the child to do as many normal things as possible.'
>
> John Collard, clinical director at Allergy UK.

- In the case of toddlers and very young children, most restaurants are happy for you to take your own snacks with you.
- Ask about everything you order. Trust your instincts – if a meal doesn't look right, send it back for the chef to check. Make it clear how dangerous mistakes can be.
- With nut allergies, it may be better if everyone at your table is also nut-free to avoid problems with any spillages.
- Get your child used to not eating certain foods when they are away from home, e.g. ice cream.
- If you have young children, you may prefer to take your own booster seat as restaurant highchairs are not usually completely clean.
- If you find one restaurant is helpful, become a regular there. Ask for the same staff and order the same food.

Birthday parties

All children love a birthday party, but food allergies, latex allergy, eczema or even dust allergy can affect their enjoyment.

- When you reply to the invitation, mention that your child has an allergy. Some parties may cause more problems than others, e.g. arts and crafts parties for children with an allergy to glue or paint.
- Children with food allergies can feel left out if they can't eat the same food as their peers. Ask what food they will be serving as you may find that your child will be able to eat some of it. If not, bring your own alternatives, e.g. nut-free chocolate spread sandwiches, dairy-free ice cream or wheat-free cakes.
- When you arrive at the party, remind the parents about your child's allergy and, in the case of food allergies, double-check the food on offer. Remember that food intended for the parents may not be suitable for your child.
- Teach your child to ask about the ingredients before they eat the party food and to only eat wrapped items they have eaten before.

- Always make sure your child has a supply of medicines with them and that they, or a responsible adult, know how to use them.
- If your child has dust allergy, remind them not to sit on the floor.
- If you are worried, stay at the party but keep in the background, or leave your child under the watchful eye of another trustworthy adult.

Sleepovers

Sleeping over at a friend's is a big step in independence, but also a big worry for parents. By the time your child is old enough to go to a sleepover, they should be ready to take some responsibility for their allergy management.

- Make the first sleepover at your house or at a good friend's house not far away. Keep the sleepovers small at first, with only two or three children.
- If your child is allergic to house dust mites, they won't be able to sleep on the floor. Their bedding needs to be clean and dust-free, so keep a spare set of anti-allergy bedding covers for sleepovers.
- Provide clear instructions for the other parents about your child's allergies and triggers, but don't worry them unnecessarily about the responsibility.
- Discuss your child's evening routine with the other parents. For example, your child may need to take their allergy medicines or apply emollients before going to bed.
- Make sure your child knows what to do if they have an allergic reaction.
- Let your child know that you are only a phone call away and make sure you can be contacted easily that evening. Don't keep checking up though – arrange to call once in the middle of the evening to check everything's okay.

Family holidays

> 'Our main aim is to stop Jessie's allergies taking over her life, but we have to assess each occasion. When her resistance is low (e.g. after an allergic reaction or a cold), she's much more sensitive and more likely to have another reaction. At these times, we are less likely to take any risks.'
>
> Gail Flaum, whose six-year-old daughter has eczema and multiple allergies (including egg, nut, chocolate and dust).

All holidays need good planning but even more so when your child has an allergy. A 'Holiday Campaign' report by Allergy UK in July 2007 found that over 50% of people have restricted their holidays because of allergies and asthma, with over 67% of people experiencing an allergic reaction while away.

There are many challenges to face in a foreign country, so some parents find it easier to holiday in Great Britain. However, all holidays can be problematic if you don't take precautions.

Plan ahead

- Ask your travel agent if any hotels can cater for people on a restricted diet. If your child has multiple or severe allergies, self-catering may be the safest option.
- Some bed and breakfasts or holiday cottages can cater for people with allergies, especially gluten or dairy. Search for suitable places on the Internet.
- Make sure you stay near medical facilities and check the locations of the nearest GPs and hospitals when you arrive.
- Some airlines operate nut-free catering policies, while others don't serve peanuts but won't stop other passengers from bringing snacks on board. Speak to the airline in advance to see what precautions they take.
- Confirm with the airline that you will be carrying adrenaline auto-injectors (EpiPens or Anapens), and get a letter from your doctor explaining why you are carrying them. You may need to show this letter at security control or check-in.
- Let the cabin crew know about your child's allergy when you arrive on the aeroplane.
- Ask your child's GP or allergy specialist about any special precautions you should take on holiday.
- Ensure that your travel insurance covers allergy treatments. Asthma UK can provide you with details of insurance plans for people with asthma. If you are travelling in the European Union, obtain a European Health Insurance Card from your local post office, or call 0845 606 2030 or visit www.ehic.org.uk.

Pack your essentials

- If you are travelling abroad, you may be able to buy a translation card to explain your child's condition in the country's native language. Translation cards are available from Allergy UK and Kidsaware. If you are travelling to a country whose language isn't covered, find a reputable translation agency to translate phrases such as 'My child is severely allergic to…'
- Pack supplies of food to eat at the airport or on the journey just in case you are delayed. Also pack some for the holiday and journey home. The less shopping you have to do while away, the better. If you do buy abroad, check the labels carefully – even well-known brands may contain different ingredients in another country and may be produced in a different factory.
- If your child has house dust mite allergy, pack anti-allergy bedding.
- Ensure you have enough medicines for your holiday plus some extra, as getting replacements may be difficult abroad. Keep the medicines out of the heat and cold and store them carefully.
- Make sure your child wears medical ID jewellery (see chapter 10) as this is an internationally recognised way of notifying foreign doctors that your child has an allergy or any medical condition.

Children's holiday camps

As your child gets older, you will want them to have the same experiences as their peers. Holiday camps and adventure holidays can give your child self-confidence and new skills, and helps them meet new friends.

Allergy camps

Asthma UK's Kick Asthma Adventure Camp is the only camp in the UK that caters especially for children with allergies, asthma or eczema. This week-long adventure holiday is supervised by fully trained volunteers and supported by healthcare professionals. It has an educational message as well as physical

> 'I don't want Jessie to grow up dwelling on what she can't do. I would prefer her to enjoy activities like playing on the sand or stroking a dog, even if we have to treat a flare up afterwards.'
>
> Gail Flaum, whose six-year-old daughter has eczema and multiple allergies (including egg, nut, chocolate and dust).

and social activities, as there are sessions on managing medicines and coping with an asthma attack. It's suitable for children from six to 17 years and is held in a variety of locations around the country throughout July and August.

For more details, call Asthma UK's Support and Information team on 08456 03 81 43 or email holidays@asthma.org.uk.

General camps

If you choose to send your child to a general residential or day camp, make sure it can cater for their needs.

- Speak to the camp about your child's allergies and medical needs before you book.
- Provide clear written instructions to all members of staff when you arrive.
- You may be able to supply your child's own food for peace of mind.
- If your child's medication requires a demonstration, get there early on the first morning to discuss it.
- From Kidsaware you can buy allergy T-shirts, stickers and bags highlighting that your child has an allergy.
- Supply your child's medication in a box clearly labelled with your child's photo and instructions.

Christmas and other family gatherings

It's easy to let your guard down at family celebrations, but not all of your relatives will understand the severity of your child's symptoms.

- Take your child's allergy medicines everywhere, even to close relatives' homes.
- Take your own treats as party foods may not be clearly labelled. Your child may also not recognise some of the foods, e.g. marzipan, which contains nuts, can look like sweets.

- If your child has latex allergy, ask about balloons and other decorations which may cause problems.
- Use an artificial Christmas tree rather than a real one because this will make it easier to avoid dust or mould.
- If your child has nut allergy, buy nut-free Christmas chocolate or Easter eggs so that they don't miss out.
- There's a risk of contamination from food on people's lips, so discourage people from kissing your child.

'It's easy to let your guard down at family celebrations, but not all of your relatives will understand the severity of your child's symptoms.'

Summing Up

- Your child should be able to join in with most family activities.
- Most restaurants will be able to cater for different allergies, but you should check first.
- Make sure your child has their medicine bag with them when they go to parties.
- Don't let your child have a sleepover until they are old enough to take some responsibility for their allergy management.
- Plan holidays carefully and well in advance.

Help List

The following charities, organisations and companies can provide information, advice, helplines and/or products relevant to children with allergies. There may be other contacts not listed here, so you should also search on the Internet for reputable contacts. The contact details were correct at the time of publication.

Allergy charities, support groups and professional organisations

Allergy UK

3 White Oak Square, London Road, Swanley, Kent, BR8 7AG
Tel: 01322 619898 (helpline)
info@allergyuk.org
www.allergyuk.org
Food intolerance website: www.foodintoleranceawareness.org
Children's allergies website: www.blossomcampaign.org
Allergy UK is the UK's leading medical charity dealing with allergies. It provides a helpline with fully trained staff, factsheets, articles, allergy alerts and product endorsement.

Anaphylaxis Campaign

PO Box 275, Farnborough, Hampshire, GU14 6SX
Tel: 01252 542029 (helpline)
info@anaphylaxis.org.uk
www.anaphylaxis.org.uk
The Anaphylaxis Campaign is a national registered charity providing support and information to people at risk of anaphylaxis (especially to foods), schools and healthcare professionals. It also issues food alerts and has an online shop.

Asthma UK

Tel: 0800 1216244 ('ask an asthma nurse')
0800 1216255 (information line, 9am-5pm, Monday to Friday)
info@asthma.org.uk

Asthma UK England
Summit House, 70 Wilson Street, London, EC2A 2DB
Tel: 020 7786 4900
info@asthma.org.uk

Asthma UK Cymru (Wales)
3rd Floor, Eastgate House, 34-43 Newport Road, Cardiff, CF24 0AB
Tel: 02920 435400
wales@asthma.org.uk

Asthma UK Scotland
4 Queen Street, Edinburgh, EH2 1JE
Tel: 01312 262544
scotland@asthma.org.uk

Asthma UK Northern Ireland
The Mount, 2 Woodstock Link, Belfast, BT6 8DD
Tel: 02890 737290
ni@asthma.org.uk
www.asthma.org.uk

Asthma UK is dedicated to helping people with asthma. The charity has a helpline, magazine, information sheets and a website. There's a forum on the website specifically for parents and carers.

British Society for Allergy and Clinical Immunology (BSACI)

Elliott House, 10/12 Allington Street, London, SW1E 5EH
Tel: 0207 8087135
www.bsaci.org

The BSACI is an organisation for healthcare professionals who work in the field of allergy. The website has a list of NHS allergy clinics for members of the public.

The British Thoracic Society (BTS)

17 Doughty Street, London, WC1N 2PL
Tel: 020 7831 8778

bts@brit-thoracic.org.uk
www.brit-thoracic.org.uk
The BTS is a registered charity with the aim of improving the standards of care for people with respiratory diseases. You can download the 2008 'British Guideline on the Management of Asthma' from the website.

European Health Insurance Card

Tel: 0845 606 2030
www.ehic-ie.org or www.ehic.org.uk
The European Health Insurance Card (formerly E111 form) is available from post offices, the telephone orderline or EHIC website.

Hyperactive Children's Support Group (HACSG)

Dept W, The Hyperactive Children's Support Group, 71 Whyke Lane, Chichester, West Sussex, PO19 7PD
Tel: 01243 539966 (this is not a helpline)
hacsg@hacsg.org.uk
www.hacsg.org.uk
The HACSG helps ADHD/hyperactive children and their families reduce or eliminate artificial food additives from their diet. For more information, send a large SAE (stamped addressed envelope) to the above address.

Latex Allergy Support Group (LASG)

PO Box 27, Filey, YO14 9YH
Tel: 07071 225838 (helpline, 7pm-10pm)
latexallergyfree@hotmail.com
www.lasg.co.uk
The LASG provides information and advice to people with latex allergy.

Medical Conditions at School Partnership

c/o Asthma UK, Summit House, 70 Wilson Street, London, EC2A 2DB
Tel: 020 7786 4900
info@asthma.org.uk
www.medicalconditionsatschool.org.uk

The Medical Conditions at School Partnership provides information for schools and school healthcare professionals to help them support all pupils with medical conditions.

National Eczema Society (NES)

Hill House, Highgate Hill, London, N19 5NA
Tel: 0800 0891122 (helpline, 8am-8pm, Monday to Friday)
helpline@eczema.org
www.eczema.org
The NES offers practical advice to people with eczema and their families and carers. The charity has a helpline, magazine for members, local support groups and information for schools and healthcare professionals.

National Pollen and Aerobiology Research Unit (NPARU)

University of Worcester, Henwick Grove, Worcester, WR2 6AJ
Tel: 01905 855200
www.pollenuk.co.uk
The NPARU conducts research into airborne allergens, such as pollen, house dust mites and moulds. Its website includes a pollen calendar and tips on avoiding exposure to pollen.

The Resuscitation Council (UK)

5th Floor, Tavistock House North, Tavistock Square, London, WC1H 9HR
Tel: 020 7388 4678
enquiries@resus.org.uk
www.resus.org.uk
The Resuscitation Council is a professional organisation for medical practitioners with an interest in the subject of resuscitation.

Medical identification (ID) jewellery

There are various companies that can supply medical identification jewellery, but the following two companies provide child-friendly products. The MedicAlert Foundation is a registered charity recommended by healthcare professionals.

ICE Gems

IdentifyMe Limited, Anani House, 2 Woodvale Road, Whitefield, Manchester, M26 1UE
Tel: 0845 1259539 or 0161 8706044 (9.30am-4.30pm, Monday to Friday)
info@identifyme.co.uk
www.icegems.co.uk
ICE (in case of emergency) wristbands have a stainless steel medical ID tag that can be engraved with your child's name and date of birth, medical condition/allergy, medication and at least one emergency contact number. The confidential information is engraved on the rear of the tag for privacy. There are no annual subscriptions or renewal fees.

The MedicAlert Foundation

1 Bridge Wharf, 156 Caledonian Road, London, N1 9UU
Tel: 0800 581420 (9am-5pm, Monday to Friday)
info@medicalert.org.uk
www.medicalert.org.uk
This non-profit making charity provides a life-saving identification system for people with hidden medical conditions and allergies. The kids' range consists of waterproof Velcro wristbands with the MedicAlert symbol on the emblem disc. Each emblem is engraved with the wearer's main medical condition/allergy or vital details, a personal ID number and a 24-hour emergency telephone number. Emergency and medical professionals can access the wearer's details (e.g. name and address, doctor's details, current drug therapy and emergency contact numbers) anywhere in the world in over 100 languages. There's an annual fee for membership plus the cost of the wristband.

Support for smokers

NHS Pregnancy Smoking Helpline

Tel: 0800 1699169
www.smokefree.nhs.uk/smoking-and-pregnancy
You can call the helpline for expert advice on the health risks of smoking during pregnancy and ways to quit.

NHS Smoking Helpline

Tel: 0800 0224332 (7.00am-11pm)
England: 0800 1690169
Northern Ireland: 0800 858585
Scotland: 0800 848484
Wales: 0300 1000 069
http://smokefree.nhs.uk

This helpline is run by the Department of Health. You can call one of the above numbers for free smoking cessation advice from a trained advisor. The website provides information on stopping smoking, nicotine replacement products and general support.

QUIT

211 Old Street, London, EC1V 9NR
Tel: 0800 002200 (quitline)
stopsmoking@quit.org.uk
www.quit.org.uk

QUIT is an independent charity set up to provide practical help, advice and support to UK smokers who wish to quit. You can consult a trained counsellor by calling or emailing the helpline. You can also buy books and leaflets through the website.

Baby feeding advice

Association of Breastfeeding Mothers (ABM)

PO Box 207, Bridgwater, Somerset, TA6 7YT
Tel: 08444 122949 (helpline)
counselling@abm.me.uk
www.abm.me.uk

The ABM was founded by a group of mothers to provide accurate information for all women wishing to breastfeed. The helpline is run by fully trained volunteer breastfeeding counsellors.

Breastfedbabies.org

Public Health Agency, Ormeau Avenue Unit, 18 Ormeau Avenue, Belfast, BT2 8HS
Tel: 02890 311611 (8.45am-5pm, Monday to Friday)
info@breastfedbabies.org
www.breastfedbabies.org
Run by the Public Health Agency for Northern Ireland, the website provides information on the benefits of breastfeeding and how to breastfeed and avoid problems. There's also a network of local breastfeeding support groups.

Breastfeeding Network

PO Box 11126, Paisley, PA2 8YB
Tel: 0300 100 0210 (supporterline)
0844 4124665 (drugs in breastmilk helpline)
breastfeeding-support-2009@breastfeedingnetworkorg.uk
www.breastfeedingnetwork.org.uk
The Breastfeeding Network provides independent breastfeeding support and advice, including information on local breastfeeding centres and taking prescription medicines while breastfeeding.

National Breastfeeding Helpline

Tel: 0300 100 0212 (helpline)
www.breastfeeding.nhs.uk
This helpline is funded by the Department of Health. It's run by trained volunteers from the Association of Breastfeeding Mothers and the Breastfeeding Network. Callers are put through to their nearest trained volunteer.

National Childbirth Trust (NCT)

Alexandra House, Oldham Terrace, London, W3 6NH
Tel: 0300 3300772 (pregnancy and birth line)
0300 3300771 (breastfeeding line)
www.nct.org.uk
The NCT is the UK's biggest parenting charity. It offers advice and information to parents during pregnancy and in the early days of parenthood. The services for parents include access to breastfeeding counsellors and local support networks.

Food and nutrition

British Dietetic Association (BDA)

5th Floor, Charles House, 148/9 Great Charles Street, Queensway, Birmingham, B3 3HT
Tel: 0121 2008080
www.bda.uk.com

This professional association provides information on the role of dietitians and factsheets on healthy eating and diet-related topics, including food allergies. You can find a dietitian through www.dietitiansunlimited.co.uk, the online search facility run by the BDA.

British Nutrition Foundation

High Holborn House, 52-54 High Holborn, London, WC1V 6RQ
Tel: 020 74046504
postbox@nutrition.org.uk
www.nutrition.org.uk

This registered charity provides information on healthy eating, nutrition and food labelling.

Food Standards Agency (FSA)

Food Standards Agency HQ and England
Aviation House, 125 Kingsway, London, WC2B 6NH
Tel: 020 72768829
helpline@foodstandards.gsi.gov.uk
www.food.gov.uk

Food Standards Agency Wales
11th Floor, South Gate House, Wood Street, Cardiff, CF10 1EW
Tel: 02920 678999
wales@foodstandards.gsi.gov.uk
www.food.gov.uk/wales

Food Standards Agency Scotland
6th Floor, St Magnus House, 25 Guild Street, Aberdeen, AB11 6NJ
Tel: 01224 285100
scotland@foodstandards.gsi.gov.uk

www.food.gov.uk/scotland
Food Standards Agency Northern Ireland
10A-C Clarendon Road, Belfast, BT1 3BG
Tel: 02890 417700
infofsani@foodstandards.gsi.gov.uk
www.food.gov.uk/northernireland
Consumer advice and information: www.eatwell.gov.uk
The FSA is an independent government agency. Its websites provide information on healthy eating, food safety, allergies and labelling. You can also receive allergy alerts via email or text.

LEAP Study

LEAP Study, Paediatric Allergy Research Department, Evelina Children's Hospital, St Thomas' Hospital, Lambeth Palace Road, London, SE1 7EH
info@leapstudy.co.uk
www.leapstudy.co.uk
The LEAP study is looking at whether peanut avoidance or peanut exposure puts children at risk of peanut allergy. The research is still in its early stages.

Allergen-free foods

Alert4allergy

www.alert4allergy.org
This service provides free email and text alerts of product recalls and other incidences where food has been wrongly labelled or contaminated with common allergens, e.g. nuts, milk, etc.

Alpro Soya

www.alprosoya.co.uk
All Alpro soya products are dairy-free and lactose-free (e.g. soya drinks and desserts).

Kinnerton Chocolate

1000 Highgate Studios, 53-79 Highgate Road, London, NW5 1TL

Tel: 020 72849503
info@kinnerton.com
www.kinnerton.com
The range includes dairy-free, nut-free, egg-free and gluten-free chocolate confectionary.

Trufree

Nutrition Point Ltd, Station Court, 442 Stockport Road, Warrington, WA4 2GW
Tel: 07041 544044 (careline, 9am-5pm, Monday to Friday)
info@trufree.co.uk
www.trufree.co.uk
The Trufree range includes wheat-free and gluten-free biscuits, crackers and snacks.

Vegan Society

Donald Watson House, 21 Hylton Street, Hockley, Birmingham, B18 6HJ
Tel: 0845 4588244 or 0121 5231730
info@vegansociety.com
www.vegansociety.com
The Vegan Society website includes egg-free and milk-free recipes. There's a section for babies and toddlers and a section on egg-substitutes.

Skincare advice and eczema products

British Association of Dermatologists (BAD)

Willan House, 4 Fitzroy Square, London, W1T 5HQ
Tel: 0207 3830266
admin@bad.org.uk
www.bad.org.uk
This is the professional organisation for British dermatologists. The BAD's website includes useful information on consulting a dermatologist, general information about the skin and factsheets on common skin diseases.

British Skin Foundation (BSF)
www.britishskinfoundation.org.uk
This registered charity raises money for skin disease research and provides information on skincare to the public.

EczemaClothing
Cotton Comfort, Unit C, Western Avenue, Matrix Park, Chorley, Lancashire, PR7 7NB
Tel: 01772 331815
enquiries@eczemaclothing.com
www.eczemaclothing.com
EczemaClothing provides pure cotton clothes and schoolwear for people with eczema, allergies and sensitive skin.

LintKids
Tel: 07884 438386
contactus@lint-kids.com
www.lint-kids.com
Lint-Kids provides 100% organic cotton schoolwear.

Allergy medicines

Anapens
Lincoln Medical Ltd, Unit 8, Wilton Business Park, Salisbury, Wiltshire, SP2 0AH
Tel: 01722 742900
www.anapen.co.uk
Lincoln Medical Ltd's website provides information on anaphylaxis and using Anapens.

EpiPens
ALK-Abello Ltd, 1 Tealgate, Hungerford, Berkshire, RG17 0YT
Tel: 01488 686016
info@uk.alk-abello.com
www.epipen.co.uk

ALK-Abello Ltd's website provides information on anaphylaxis and using EpiPens, as well as an Expiry Alert Service. You can also sign up for a free trainer pen and leaflet pack.

Allergy awareness products

Allergy & Intolerance Resources

PO Box 836, Taunton, Somerset, TA4 3WS
Tel: 0871 2002309
info@go2air.co.uk
www.go2air.co.uk
This company can provide various products, including AllergyChums (stickers, clothing and wristbands) and Chef-Notes (pre-printed jotter pad sheets to fill in for restaurants notifying them of your allergy).

Kidsaware

PO Box 115, Bedford, MK44 2FA
Tel: 08702 202452
sales@kidsaware.co.uk and info@kidsaware.co.uk
www.kidsaware.co.uk
Kidsaware provides products to highlight allergic children's dietary needs. The range includes labels, stickers, carry cases, bags, wristbands, clothing and translation cards.

Yellow Cross

PO Box 448, Farnham, Surrey, GU9 8ZU.
Tel: 01252 820321
www.yellowcross.co.uk
Yellow Cross provides medical bags for adults and children, personal ID tags, translation cards and tough tubes for EpiPens.

Complementary therapy organisations

Aromatherapy Council (AC)
www.aromatherapycouncil.co.uk
This governing body for the UK aromatherapy profession can advise on recognised qualifications and professional membership associations.

British Acupuncture Council
63 Jeddo Road, London, W12 9HQ
Tel: 020 8735 0400
info@acupuncture.org.uk
www.acupuncture.org.uk
This represents professional acupuncturists in the UK and guarantees safe practice and ethical behaviour.

British Association for Applied Nutrition and Nutritional Therapy (BANT)
Tel: 08706 061284
theadministrator@bant.org.uk
www.bant.org.uk
The BANT website has the facility to search for a local nutritional therapist.

British Homeopathic Association
Hahnemann House, 29 Park Street West, Luton, LU1 3BE
Tel: 01582 408675
info@britishhomeopathic.org
www.trusthomeopathy.org
This promotes homeopathy practised by doctors and other healthcare professionals, e.g. pharmacists.

British Medical Acupuncture Society (BMAS)
Northwich office: BMAS House, 3 Winnington Court, Northwich, Cheshire, CW8 1AQ
Tel: 01606 786782

admin@medical-acupuncture.org.uk
London office: BMAS, Royal London Homoeopathic Hospital, 60 Great Ormond Street, London, WC1N 3HR
Tel: 020 77139437
bmaslondon@aol.com
www.medical-acupuncture.co.uk
This charity encourages the use and understanding of acupuncture. BMAS members are all healthcare professionals, e.g. GPs.

Buteyko Breathing Association

15 Stanley Place, Chipping Ongar, Essex, CM5 9SU
Tel: 01277 366906
info@buteykobreathing.org
www.buteykobreathing.org
This non profitmaking organisation is committed to improving the health of asthmatics and people with other breathing-related problems. Practitioners have a code of conduct.

International Federation of Professional Aromatherapists (IFPA)

82 Ashby Road, Hinckley, Leicestershire, LE10 1SN
Tel: 01455 637987
admin@ifparoma.org
www.ifparoma.org
This organisation maintains a register of practising members and maintains codes of ethics and conduct.

National Institute of Medical Herbalists

Elm House, 54 Mary Arches Street, Exeter, EX4 3BA
Tel: 01392 426022
info@nimh.org.uk
www.nimh.org.uk
This professional body represents medical herbalists.

Nutritional Therapy Council

PO Box 6114, Bournemouth, BH1 9BL
Tel: 01425 462507

info@nutrionaltherapycouncil.co.uk
www.nutritionaltherapycouncil.org.uk
This regulatory body for practitioners can confirm whether a practitioner is registered if you know their name.

The Prince's Foundation for Integrated Health
PO Box 65104, London, SW1P 9PJ
Tel: 020 7024 5755
contactus@fih.org.uk
www.fih.org.uk
Launched by HRH the Prince of Wales in 1993, this charity promotes integrated healthcare. The website includes information on healthy living and complementary therapies.

Register of Chinese Herbal Medicine (RCHM)
Office 5, 1 Exeter Street, Norwich, NR2 4QB
Tel: 01603 623994
herbmed@rchm.co.uk
www.rchm.co.uk
The RCHM regulates the practice of Chinese herbal medicine in the UK and helps members of the public find a properly qualified practitioner.

Society of Homeopaths
11 Brookfield, Duncan Close, Moulton Park, Northampton, NN3 6WL
Tel: 0845 4506611
info@homeopathy.soh.org
www.homeopathy-soh.org
This society represents professional homeopaths and can provide a register of those trained.

Need - 2 - Know

Available Titles Include ...

Allergies A Parent's Guide
ISBN 978-1-86144-064-8 £8.99

Autism A Parent's Guide
ISBN 978-1-86144-069-3 £8.99

Drugs A Parent's Guide
ISBN 978-1-86144-043-3 £8.99

Dyslexia and Other Learning Difficulties
A Parent's Guide ISBN 978-1-86144-042-6 £8.99

Bullying A Parent's Guide
ISBN 978-1-86144-044-0 £8.99

Epilepsy The Essential Guide
ISBN 978-1-86144-063-1 £8.99

Teenage Pregnancy The Essential Guide
ISBN 978-1-86144-046-4 £8.99

Gap Years The Essential Guide
ISBN 978-1-86144-079-2 £8.99

How to Pass Exams A Parent's Guide
ISBN 978-1-86144-047-1 £8.99

Child Obesity A Parent's Guide
ISBN 978-1-86144-049-5 £8.99

Applying to University The Essential Guide
ISBN 978-1-86144-052-5 £8.99

ADHD The Essential Guide
ISBN 978-1-86144-060-0 £8.99

Student Cookbook - Healthy Eating The Essential Guide
ISBN 978-1-86144-061-7 £8.99

Stress The Essential Guide
ISBN 978-1-86144-054-9 £8.99

Adoption and Fostering A Parent's Guide
ISBN 978-1-86144-056-3 £8.99

Special Educational Needs A Parent's Guide
ISBN 978-1-86144-057-0 £8.99

The Pill An Essential Guide
ISBN 978-1-86144-058-7 £8.99

University A Survival Guide
ISBN 978-1-86144-072-3 £8.99

Diabetes The Essential Guide
ISBN 978-1-86144-059-4 £8.99

View the full range at **www.need2knowbooks.co.uk**. To order our titles, call **01733 898103**, email **sales@n2kbooks.com** or visit the website.

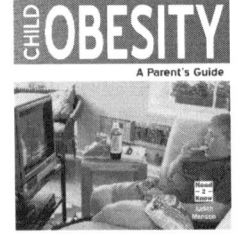

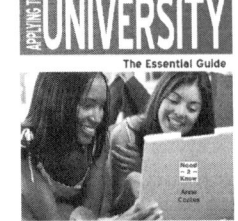

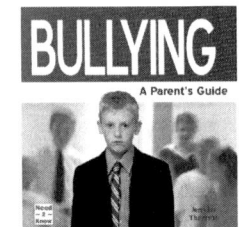

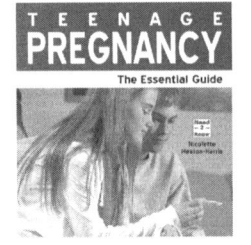

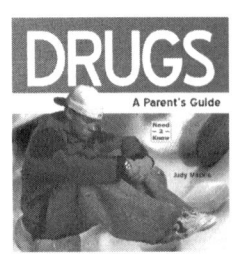

Need - 2 - Know, Remus House, Coltsfoot Drive, Peterborough, PE2 9JX